D1722693

REBOOTING THE BIOME

HOW PROPERLY CARING FOR YOUR **SKIN BIOME** CAN DO MORE FOR YOUR **HEALTH AND BEAUTY** THAN ANY SKINCARE INGREDIENT ON THE MARKET

DORIS DAY, M.D. AND
THOMAS M. HITCHCOCK, PH.D.

Prominence Publishing, www.prominencepublishing.com.

Rebooting the Biome/ Day, Doris, M.D. and Hitchcock, Thomas M., Ph.D. -- 1st ed.

ISBN: 978-1-990830-21-1

Table of Contents

PART I
RELEARNING THE BIOME

CHAPTER 1

ECOSYSTEM EQUILIBRIUM

If you don't like bacteria, you're on the wrong planet.
—Stewart Brand

Imagine you are slowly walking across an open field. As a gentle breeze blows across your cheeks, you look down to see that the field is lined with lush, green grass that is high enough to brush your knees as you wade forward. Peeking through the grass, you see a smattering of wildflowers and flowering bushes, their colors vivid and alluring. Looking around, you notice that the field is framed with leafy deciduous trees, their branches gently moving back and forth in the late spring breeze. As you feel the breeze softly hit your face you stop, close your eyes and listen. Along with the sound of the wind, you can hear the songs of the birds and the buzz of insects as they hurry past you to fulfill their daily duties. Reopening your eyes, you can see movement in the grass and the bushes as critters forage for food and make their way back to the tree line where they have made their homes. You hear the cry of the eagle above you and the babbling of a distant brook. Life is all around you. You can see it. You can hear it. You can feel it. You begin to contemplate whether you really know how *much* life is around you? A dozen species? A hundred? More? No sooner does this thought cross your mind when you hear the howl of a wolf behind you.

You turn to see that a pack of grey wolves, at least a dozen, have emerged from the tree line. Taken off guard, you stand perfectly still, hoping to avoid detection. However, the attention of one unusually large wolf falls upon you. As it stares at you, you begin to sweat. Eventually another and then another fixes their gaze on you until all of them are looking *right at you*. The large one takes a slow but deliberate step in your direction, causing your heart and mind to race as you contemplate when will be a good time to make a run for it. But before you can move, for no apparent reason their attention shifts. They all look away and begin to retreat quickly into the woods until they are all gone from sight, and you are left with a very different feeling about the life around you than before they appeared.

Now let's come back to reality and take a moment to assess what just transpired. How did you feel in the brief fantasy? Did the entrance of the wolves in your serene surroundings change the way you saw the ecosystem? Would you change it if you could; perhaps remove the wolves (humanely, of course) but keep the rest? After all, it was quite nice until they arrived, wasn't it?

As ideal as that sounds in our fantasy, in our reality it poses an interesting dilemma. At times, humans have tried to change ecosystems according to their preferences, only to find that adding or removing any given species can create major unwanted repercussions. For example, in the early 1900s the US government sanctioned hunting of "troublesome" grey wolves that were preying on the livestock of settlers of Yellowstone National Park. The plan was to outright eradicate them to make it safer for further settlement and agriculture. The plan worked, and the wolves were eliminated from the park by 1926, but the impact that followed was completely unexpected and devastating. The land fell into a deplorable condition, caused mainly by the now unchecked and rampant growth in the elk population. There were no longer any wolves to help control their numbers. With the increase in elk, there was now overgrazing of foliage that had previously served to curb erosion, provide shade to waterways, supply other animals with food such as berries, and give leaves, bark, twigs, roots, and aquatic plants for smaller species such as beavers. As foliage became scarcer, erosion rapidly increased. The habitats for beavers, grizzlies, waterfowl, wading birds, otters, moose, fish, amphibians, and more began to diminish, as did the numbers of those species. The whole ecosystem was in disarray, all because one element—the grey wolf—was removed.

The happy ending is that when wolves were eventually reintroduced to Yellowstone Park in 1995, the ecosystem began to repair itself. Perhaps some irony to be found there. The takeaway is that there are going to be some sort of repercussions to any significant change to any ecosystem, and the extent of repercussions depend on:

1. What the change is (i.e., what species, how fast the species reproduces)

2. What role the species plays in the ecosystem (i.e., is it a key predator or food source)

3. Whether the species is redundant in its role (i.e., another species can take its place in the food chain)

4. How much change happens at once (i.e., kill ten grey wolves versus kill *all* grey wolves)

There is also the way human habitation and industrialization are known to affect certain ecosystems, but we won't dwell on that here since it is far too political and divergent for this book's focus. Regardless, the world has an array of different ecosystems, and they all have some sort of balance—at least until something significant changes, whether caused by man or by nature.

Let's now make this very personal. You would be hard pressed to find any ecosystem on the planet, even your own body, that isn't teeming with bacteria. While there are tens of thousands of known, named species of bacteria, it has been recently hypothesized that 99.999% of bacteria species are yet to be discovered and named. And just like grey wolves, beavers, and humans, microorganisms such as bacteria require a specific balance in their ecosystems in order to survive and thrive. Certain species of bacteria grow best—or perhaps die—in a given ecosystem, depending on the available food source, the temperature, the other species of microbes that live there, and so on. That's all very similar to the requirements of larger multicellular species, like wolves and elk, and their ideal habitats.

And wouldn't you know it, some species of bacteria seem to consider the human body their perfect ecosystem. Thus, from birth to the grave, our bodies house billions or more likely trillions of microbes. Yet, when it comes to the human body, there are many ecosystems within it. After all, the conditions on your face are not the same as those in your bowels— one would hope. An organ such as your skin is made up of more than just the structural proteins of collagen and elastin. It has more than just the cellular layers of the epidermis and the dermis. The structure of your skin houses an entire ecosystem made up of both the human parts and the billions of microorganisms that are completely invisible to the human eye. The population of this ecosystem goes far beyond the skin's surface; it thrives deep within and throughout all its layers. And despite our often ill-advised attempts to rid ourselves of these miniscule creatures (like what we attempted to do with the grey wolf), we are learning more and more that their presence not only serves a purpose but is also linked to our health. We are inextricably linked to this tiny but vital mixture of bacteria, fungi, viruses, and archaea that we call **the microbiome**. Together with our respective microbiomes, we make up an ecosystem we call the human biome. And more specifically, the ecosystems (yes, there are multiple) contained within the many areas of skin would collectively be called the skin biome.

So, does our skin biome require the same type of balance that ecosystems such as Yellowstone National Park require? Can adding or removing the wrong microbes cause an imbalance that leads to biological disaster? Let us explore.

The Road to Dysbiosis is Paved with Good Intentions

Dr. Hitchcock: I love microbes. I have spent the better part of my life studying them in some capacity. When others have reeled in disgust at the thought of a fecal transplant or how the skin is constantly teeming with microbes no matter how much we try to wash them off, I have always found it fascinating. I find microbes so amazing that my motto for the better part of a decade has been this: "There are billions of bacteria on your face, and I think that's awesome!" However, there was a brief time when I did not feel that way because I was lying in a hospital room, feverish, emaciated, and nearly dead—all because of bacteria (I thought). Let me give you a bit of context.

As if my post-doctoral education was not difficult enough, one day when I was in the last year of my training, I noticed that a lump on my skin had begun to hurt. I was young and thought myself invincible, so I ignored it for a while as I was a poor student and did not want to incur unnecessary medical expenses—that is, until it started to burn and throb badly enough, so I knew I needed help. Assuming I probably had an infection, I went to the clinic where the doctors examined me briefly and promptly wrote a prescription for an antibiotic. For whatever reason, they made no attempt to take any cultures to find out what kind of infection I had, so I assumed they had it under control and knew exactly what they were doing. I filled the prescription and started the antibiotics course, expecting prompt relief.

What I experienced was the opposite of relief. Three days into the antibiotic series the infection had progressed to a state where I was in agony. I went back to the clinic, and a doctor told me I had an abscess and that I needed to head to the ER to have it taken care of promptly. At that point I was so miserable that I was ready to try anything. Little did I know what was to come. I won't go into all the gruesome details, but the procedure required was the most painful thing I had ever experienced, even to this day. As they proceeded to cut into my skin (yes, they had to take a chunk out) I white-knuckled the table with all my might to avoid yelling in pain. I must have asked the surgeons "are you done?" at least a dozen times in the span of the five minutes it took to complete the procedure. It was the longest . . . five . . . minutes . . . ever! Afterward, they packed the wound, sent me home, and told me to stop taking the antibiotics. Though I thought stopping the antibiotics was a weird call since I now had a large wound, I complied, believing that the surgeons knew what they were doing.

Wrong again. The doses of strong antibiotics they had initially given me had already started killing some of the bacteria in and on my body, and the incomplete course left me vulnerable. Without my good bacteria to defend me, I ended up with a nasty case of Clostridium difficile (C. difficile), a microbe that many people have in their GI tract without issue since they typically have other good bacteria to keep it in check. Within twelve hours of the surgery (and now without my good bacteria), the C. difficile grew unchecked, wreaking havoc on my GI tract and leaving me severely dehydrated and exhausted to the point that I couldn't even stand. Now I was both sick and scared. Out of desperation I called my father who drove six hours to pick me up off the floor and help me get to the emergency room.

At the ER, doctors told me that I not only had a C. difficile infection but also a Staph infection—and not just any Staph infection but a Methicillin-resistant Staphylococcus aureus (MRSA) infection to boot. I most likely acquired it from the hospital while my immune system was busy fighting C. difficile. Since MRSA (and C. difficile) is an opportunistic infection that can be lethal, I was hospitalized in a private room (silver lining?) where visitors could only come in if they wore gowns, gloves, and masks. And if that wasn't enough, I also came down with hospital-acquired pneumonia. Finally, after a couple weeks and some strong antibiotics by IV to clean up the mess, I was discharged from the hospital—20 pounds lighter and furious at the mistakes I felt the physicians made that could have killed me. But ultimately, I was happy to be alive and well again. That is when I began truly to respect the important balance in our microbiomes and how much more careful thought and consideration should be given when using systemic, microbiome-altering antibiotics.

GERMS ARE BAD, RIGHT?

Given the bad publicity that microbes have received over the last century or so, it's no wonder people overreact to them, and over sanitize themselves. Due to the viral pandemic that began in 2019, the level of anxiety over germs is understandably at an all-time high for many people. During that period, the media made many of us feel like we're all just one sneeze or cough droplet away from getting very, very sick or dying. Everywhere we looked, we saw warnings to wash your hands, use hand sanitizer, wear a face covering, and beware of the person coughing next to you. Who among us didn't experience the agony of holding in an innocent cough just to avoid "the look"? It was even worse if you had to travel or got stuck in a crowded space like an elevator or airplane.

Fear of microbes is the reason we wash our hands before we eat and after we use the bathroom. It's also the reason it's polite (and now fully expected) to cover your mouth when you sneeze or cough. It's the reason a nurse cleans your skin with alcohol wipes before an injection and why surgeons wear sterile garments and gloves to operate. It's the reason microbe-destroying ingredients are added to soaps, wipes, cleansers, and sanitizers—the ones we have been conditioned to feel we *must* use or we'll put ourselves at greater risk for getting sick—or even dying.

Regardless, microbes—especially bacteria—are inescapable. As you walk across a room, you are literally wading through a sea of microbes. When you sleep, you are sleeping with billions of microbes. When you eat, you are consuming microbes. So, if microbes all cause disease, why aren't we all sick more often if not all the time?

The answer is that the relationship between germs and the human body is much more complicated than we originally thought.

JUDGE NOT YOUR GERMS

According to the Merriam-Webster dictionary, a germ is "a micro-organism causing disease: a pathogenic agent (such as a bacterium or virus); broadly: microorganism."

According to this definition, a germ has two attributes. First, it's a microorganism (also referred to as a microbe). Second, it is pathogenic (meaning it causes disease). So, for a germ to be considered a germ, it must be *both* a microorganism and pathogenic, as you can see in this Venn diagram. To put it simply, by this interpretation of the definition, all germs are microbes, but not all microbes are germs.

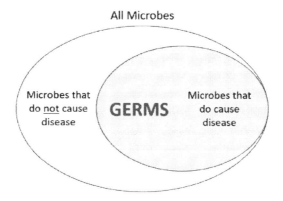

Of course, it is never that simple. If we do a bit of mental gymnastics, we can derive another way to interpret the dictionary definition of a germ. Rather than a germ being a microbe *and* pathogenic, what if we think of a germ as a microbe that's *acting* pathogenic? An analogy of this would be a dog, let's say a beagle, that lives in a household where people have allergies to dogs. That would be problematic. However, in a household where nobody is allergic to dogs, the beagle would be *the best dog ever*. So whether or not the dog is considered a problem is relative to the situation. In the same way, a microbe that might be pathogenic in some environments or under some circumstances may not be pathogenic in other environments and circumstances. Thus, calling a microbe a germ when it is only conditionally pathogenic leads to confusion, and rightfully so. To take that one step further, some microbes have situations or strains where they can behave better or worse. Think of a dog that needs training so he knows to wait for his walk to relieve himself. We'll cover this in greater detail as it relates to microbes when we talk about how microbes relate to skin diseases in Chapter 4.

So a particular microbe could sometimes, but not always, fit the definition of a germ. What we are learning is that it is partially a balancing act and partially dependent on features of the microbe itself. Some microbes that are considered germs have long been thought to cause disease but are now known to be commensal (provide neither benefit nor disease) or even symbiotic (provide benefit) in nature. In this context, what could be considered bad (i.e., a germ) could also be considered good (a symbiote). Also, some germs that cause opportunistic infections in immune-compromised individuals can live in or on another body without any known health implications.

An example of this is *Staphylococcus epidermidis*, which is thought to be a skin commensal (doesn't cause harm normally) but is also one of the most common causes for hospital-acquired infections. When we start to understand the complexity of the interaction of microbes with the human body, the definition of a germ becomes a bit reductive and moot. That is why we don't use the word *germ* in this book in reference to microbes in general. Instead, we use the term *microbe* generically or state the exact type (e.g., bacterium, fungus, archaea, virus) as appropriate.

Now that we have a clearer understanding of what we are working with, let's take a closer look at the specific microbes that arguably make up the vast majority of the body's microbiome—bacteria.

UBIQUITOUS BACTERIA

If the 3.5-billion-year-old fossil records are to be believed, bacteria appeared on this planet eons before humans. Yet given their assumed age, bacteria are not only still here in vast amounts, but due to their persistence, resilience, and adaptiveness, they're likely to outlive most species of creatures long after we depart. They even clean up after us when we do depart; microbes are a key component of the decomposition of the body upon death. Yes, teeming hordes of bacteria are always on, around, and in us from birth till death.

Scientists have found bacteria in the deepest parts of the ocean and as high as 40 miles into the atmosphere. We are still discovering new species in the most unusual places. Because bacteria are so numerous and ubiquitous, there is no way to quantify how many actually exist in nature—any guess would probably be too conservative, but it has been estimated that there are somewhere in the ballpark of 500 octillion bacteria on earth (that's *thirty* zeros). That's 100 million times greater than all the stars in the known universe. Clorox wipes aren't going to make a dent.

We know for sure that there are a lot of bacteria, but despite their vast numbers, they are so small that they went undiscovered for most of human history. Although they are tiny, they can be formidable. Many of them can harm or kill you under the right circumstances. However (and this is of the highest importance) there are also many that are beneficial, even vital, to health and life, especially on your skin, your body's largest organ and its primary contact with our world.

There is a complexity in the relationship between our human cells and the cells of the skin microbiome that we still have much to learn about. Species of bacteria we once may have feared might *actually* be made up of dozens of subspecies (or strains) that are critical to the health of the skin – discussed in Chapter 3. Others, of course, may contribute to disease. So when it comes to the microbiome and our health, it is not as simple as labeling these "germs" good or bad. We're learning that it may not simply be the presence of one species of microbe that causes disease; it could also be the *absence* of one or more species that is a more relevant factor (or maybe both). We'll discuss this in Chapter 4. We're also learning that our immune system not only plays a role in protecting us from certain microbes but can be influenced by them as well. Yes, some microbes can be a bad influence on you (science humor, not sorry).

As scientists first learned about the potential for some microbes to be associated with disease, they tried to find ways to attempt to sterilize the skin. Antibiotics, antimicrobials, and preservatives are a means to curb the growth of what they saw as germs and are now found in nearly all our skin care and personal hygiene products. While there may have been sound reasoning for that when bacteria were thought to all be bad, we now realize that it isn't necessarily a good thing for many skin products and medicines to be antimicrobial. Some of the antimicrobial habits we've gotten used to are, in reality, counterproductive. It's like trying to eradicate more than the grey wolves in Yellowstone…it's like trying to eradicate many species in Yellowstone. Within that category of so-called germs that antibacterial ingredients are set to kill are those species that specifically play a major role in the upkeep of the health, functionality, and even beauty of your skin. In case we haven't made it perfectly clear, this means that trying to have as sterile skin as possible may end up doing you more harm than good.

MEET YOUR AMAZING MICROBES

The human eye can see things that are around one-tenth of a millimeter. That's pretty small. Most microorganisms are about one-tenth that size. Just so you know how tiny bacteria are, a single Staphylococcus bacterium cell is about 1 μm by 1 μm in size. That's *one-millionth* of a meter. It's so tiny that hundreds of thousands of these little creatures could fit comfortably in the period at the end of this sentence. Viruses are even more miniscule—about 100 times smaller. It wasn't until the electron microscope was invented in the 1930s that scientists were able to see them at all.

Dr. Hitchcock: When I began studying microbiology in college, my first project was with the common red bread mold, Neurospora crassa. What we see as a fuzzy coating on rotting food is actually an intricate web of filaments and reproductive structures. This gave me a peek into the world of the microbiome where things seen by the naked eye did not always translate into the intricacy of what was happening in each microcosm. While this was a great first foray into the microbiome, it wasn't until I started my doctoral work in genetics at Clemson University that my eyes were fully opened to the astonishing universe of microbes, especially a bacterium called Deinococcus radiodurans. You've likely never heard of it, but it's actually listed in the Guinness Book of World Records as "the world's toughest bacteria." Known as polyextremophile—meaning it can survive in a number of truly harsh environments—this little bacterium can persist despite extreme cold, dehydration, vacuum, and acids, and is one of the most radiation-resistant organisms in the world (thus the name radiodurans, the Latin radius and durare, meaning "radiation surviving"). You can literally shatter its DNA, and it's able to piece it back together and thrive. How does something we consider so primitive do this while we humans cannot? It's something to think about.

The human microbiota is diverse and includes bacteria, viruses, and eukaryotes such as fungi, helminths, and protozoa. In this book, we're concentrating on your skin's microbiome and focusing even further on the bacterial part of the microbiome, the largest and most studied component. But it's important for you to know about the other kinds of microbes, especially since so many people get understandably confused about their differences.

Bacteria

Bacteria are single-celled microorganisms. They have cell walls but lack organelles and an organized nucleus, and thus are called prokaryotes (eukaryotes are cells with a nucleus). As far as we currently know, these microbes make up the vast majority of the skin microbiome.

Archaea

Archaea are single-celled microorganisms that are also classified as prokaryotes since they have much of the same physical characteristics as bacteria. For a while, they were considered a type of bacteria. However, they are a distinct domain of organism with certain attributes more like bacteria and certain attributes more like eukaryotes (such as fungus). While archaea do not have any disease association, not much is known about them regarding the skin microbiome other than they play an insignificant role (we think). One interesting study showed that the older you are, the more archaea you have on your skin—what that means for our skin health is TBD.

Viruses

Viruses are the smallest of the microbes (the known ones at least) and are not considered a prokaryote despite not having a nucleus. In fact, viruses are not even *living* entities. They typically consist of genetic material (DNA or RNA) and maybe some proteins packaged in a type of shell used to deliver the contents into the target cells. Viruses can't survive on their own and can multiply only by hijacking a living cell. While the virobiome (viruses in the microbiome as a whole) is not well-studied, it could have a large impact on the health of human skin since most of the skin virobiome is made up of bacteriophages—viruses that don't infect human cells but only infect the bacteria of the microbiome.

Fungi

Fungi are the first kind of eukaryotic microbes in the microbiome. Like the virobiome, the fungus part of the microbiome has its own name— the mycobiome. Types of microbes in this classification include yeasts and molds. Although most people think of the familiar mushroom when they think of fungi, mushrooms do not exist in the skin microbiome.

Some fungi can live on the skin without any issues; however, overgrowth or imbalance can lead to issues such as acne and dermatitis (discussed in Chapter 4).

Protozoa and Helminths

Okay, we don't really hear much about these guys—protozoa and helminths—when reading about the microbiome, but we will give you just a taste. They are present and are technically microbes. Protozoa are a group of single-celled eukaryotes, either free-living or parasitic, that feed on organic matter such as other microorganisms or organic tissues and debris. Helminths are microscopic worms. While these organisms can live in the gastrointestinal tract of humans (mostly in third world countries), their infestation or infection is usually associated with disease. It is possible, though, that these organisms may have some part to play in the balance of the body's overall microbiome, but little is known about whether either of these types of microbes have any role in the skin microbiome.

So we have at least four or five types of microbes in the skin microbiome, and bacteria are the most prevalent by far. With billions of microbes all over our skin—different domains, species, and strains—how do we know which ones help us and which ones hurt us?

THE HOLOBIONT PHILOSOPHY

We are living in a microbial renaissance of sorts. That's because science is now able to look inside the world of the microbiome with more clarity and resolution than ever before. It is deepening our understanding of how the microbes in and on our bodies truly interact with our human cells and what that means for the health and beauty of our skin.

In large part, that is due to cutting-edge technologies such as 16S rRNA sequencing. We won't get into the technical description of what 16S rRNA sequencing is in this book; all you need to know is that it is a quick and accurate way to determine all the bacteria in any given sample, even down to the different strains. Before this amazing development, scientists were dependent on culturing bacteria and seeing what appeared on a Petri dish. As it has been estimated that about 1% of bacteria are culturable, this left scientists with a very small piece of the picture. Now we can identify the vast majority—if not all—of the known bacteria in any given place on the body, not just the ones we're able to culture in the lab. We are finding bacteria species and strains (subspecies) we didn't even know existed, which is allowing scientists to start collecting vast amounts of data about the types of bacteria that live on the skin and whether they can be linked to several factors such as age, diet, gender, and disease.

That brings us back to the beginning of this chapter. Like the grey wolves in Yellowstone National Park, there is an ecological balance that needs to be achieved between us as human hosts (the environment) and our microbiomes (the "little animals" that inhabit us). If we fail to achieve this balance, just like in Yellowstone we can end up with an imbalance that can lead to skin issues or even systemic issues. But to reach a balance, in today's world, a change in philosophy must occur—recognizing that by caring for the whole ecosystem (the holobiont or "whole of the biomes"), we are able to *best* care for ourselves. By now you realize that our prolific prokaryote friends—bacteria—are ubiquitous and make up a large part of our microbiomes. Our skin, while protective in design, is not an impenetrable barrier; we now know that bacteria live not only on the surface of our skin but also deep inside us as well. Many of the microorganisms that reside in and on the skin also provide vital functions that your body can't perform on its own. Although there are some bad actors in the microbiome that can harm us, it isn't as simple as "germs cause disease." To best serve ourselves, we need to better understand our microbes and their relationship to our bodies as their ecosystems. In doing so, it *is* possible to achieve a symbiotic interaction with these microbes to help keep us alive, well, and beautiful.

CHAPTER 2

MARRIED TO THE MICROBE

The role of the infinitely small in nature is infinitely great.
—Louis Pasteur

The marriage between humans and microbes has always been precarious. When things are good, we don't notice they are there, and we certainly don't think about the good they may be doing for us. Yet there have been many times when the relationship has gone awry. You might assume that this is the fault of the microbes, and often you would be correct (after all, microbes sometimes have boundary issues). However, you must admit that humans don't appreciate their microbes the way they should, and they can be a bit overreactive and at times outright hostile to the microbes when misunderstandings arise. All it takes is a slightly inflammatory issue caused by a few bad microbe actors, and humans basically throw the proverbial A-bomb (antibiotics) at the whole darn microbiome. Microbial genocide ensues, leaving the door open for microbial retribution. The back and forth can seem relentless, and in the end, the damage is often more than hurt feelings. It is a mess of a microbe-human marriage. Like any tough relationship, you might sometimes wonder, "would I be better off alone? Do I really *need* them?" And the answer to that is a definitive *yes* . . . and *no*…but really *yes*.

That's correct, let us explain.

It seems that we don't *need* our microbes to stay alive (well, not technically at least), and the evidence for this lies in a humanmade curiosity we call germ-free animals. These animals are exactly what their moniker suggests; they are cultivated to be free of any and all microbes—

sterile, if you will—both inside and out. Given that pretty much every nook and cranny of the earth is teeming with microbes, you may appreciate how difficult arranging such a thing might be. In the post-World War II 1940s, the development of this very concept became a reality at the University of Notre Dame where scientists used research by James Arthur Reyniers and Philip Charles Trexler. Their research is not for the faint of heart or for animal lovers. The creation of the first germ-free animal was done methodically by sacrificing the mother right before she gave birth, sterilizing the freshly deceased body, and immediately removing the intact uterus that held the offspring. It was placed in a germ-free surgical isolator (an incubator of sorts), and then the uterus was disinfected through various procedures such as dunking it into antiseptics prior to releasing the offspring and putting it into another sterile incubator.[1] For the remainder of their days, these animals would then live in isolation, without direct contact from other animals, unless being used in an experiment or if they were to be bred in sterile environments to keep the germ-free lines going. While that process sounds (and may be) a bit brutal, it did eventually prove successful to produce animals that did not have any microorganisms in their bodies—well, at least none that could be detected. While it was always possible that there could be some tiny amounts of undetectable microbial contamination in these animals, it was generally assumed they were essentially microbe-free.

But what do these animals teach us about our dependence on or independence from our microbes? To answer that, we should first look even farther back in history to see why scientists ventured to even make such animals.

ANTI-*CULTURE* CULTURE

The idea that the world could someday be free of microbes became prominent in the late 1800s, as outlined by Robert Kirk in a review of this era. The question of whether bacteria were either *critical for* or *detrimental to* life became a topic of controversy among scientists. During that time, even noteworthy microbiologist Louis Pasteur posed the question of whether such experimentation was ethical or even necessary. He did this publicly when he called out his colleague and friend Émile Duclaux who had begun to focus her research on "pure cultures" of plants that were cultivated in isolation from microorganisms. The intention was that bacteria were bad for the development of most organisms and that by getting rid of microbes, we would all be free of disease.[2] In stark contrast, Pasteur believed that many bacteria were absolutely critical to the function of more complex organisms. That might seem counter to the work Pasteur is most known for—making advances in health through the discovery of the principles of vaccination and pasteurization, both aiming to remove select microbes from humans. Yet even at this time when the science of microbiology was still in its infancy, Pasteur realized that while some bacteria are detrimental, not all are, and he believed it was shortsighted and foolish for anyone, scientist or not, to assume that they are.

This debate even found its way into popular culture. One of the most famous examples is H. G. Wells' 1898 novel *The War of the Worlds* where earth is invaded by Martians who seek to eradicate humans and claim the world for themselves, only to fail quite suddenly in the eleventh hour as they succumb unsuspectingly to infections from the many microbes found on earth. The final passage reads like this:

For so it had come about, as indeed I and many men might have foreseen had not terror and disaster blinded our minds. These germs of disease have taken toll of humanity since the beginning of things—taken toll of our prehuman ancestors since life began here. But by virtue of this natural selection of our kind we have developed resisting power; to no germs do we succumb without a struggle, and to many—those that cause putrefaction in dead matter, for instance—our living frames are altogether immune. But there are no bacteria in Mars, and directly these invaders arrived, directly they drank and fed, our microscopic allies began to work their overthrow. Already when I watched them, they were irrevocably doomed, dying and rotting even as they went to and fro. It was inevitable. By the toll of a billion deaths man has bought his birthright of the earth, and it is his against all comers; it would still be his were the Martians ten times as mighty as they are. For neither do men live nor die in vain.[3]

Essentially, humans were saved in the end due to the balance they had achieved with earth's microbes over the millennia, but the aliens had not achieved such immunity—an oversight that cost them the war. While the sentiment of such fantastical literature agreed with Pasteur and though the scientific community seemed to applaud Wells' accuracy in his depiction of the essential balance between microbes and humans, the sentiment would not be sustained long into the new century.[4] Perhaps because the layperson vehicle of the sentiment was science fiction, it unknowingly led the public to believe it may not be scientific fact.

Despite the misgivings of Pasteur and many other scientists, the germ-free-is-better sentiment began to propagate, in large part due to the culture of the day. Even though antibiotics were yet to be discovered, it was well entrenched in the American and European cultures as early as the 1910s that germ-free living was going to be a large part of a much-anticipated utopian future. There was a shift in the perspectives of the literature of the time where novels and magazines spun fantastic and futuristic tales of how the world would be in centuries to come when it rid itself of microbial contaminations and people live in utter bliss. These fictional narratives that propagated such concepts did not simply come from the minds of creative authors; they were inspired by headlines of the prior decade.

In 1914, claims by prominent scientists such as Ilya Mechnikov and Michel Cohendy to have produced germ-free chickens and guinea pigs were blasted across the pages of the *New York Times*, touting that a germ-free existence was possible.[5,6] While there was indeed much skepticism from many scientists about the methods used to create and sustain the alleged germ-free environments (since it had not yet been optimized or substantiated by Arthur and Trexler), that did not stop the idea from becoming firmly planted in the American psyche. After all, when Cohendy made claims that his supposed germ-free chickens grew faster and larger than other chickens, the *New York Times* published headlines that this would be possible for children as well. And we wonder where the first world obsession with overcleanliness came from?

Once the 1940s arrived and the creation of the first verifiably germ-free animals took place, it emboldened those with the sentiment that a sterile world would be better for all. Scientists keenly observed germ-free animals to see if this emerging philosophy was indeed the wave of the future as they debated whether science would meet the fiction from the decades prior. The debate extended for decades as noteworthy scientists continued to speculate on the possibilities of a sterile world.

One debate was captured by acclaimed virologist Hilary Koprowski in his 1963 publication "Man and His Future" where he recalls a disagreement between him and Nobel Prize winning molecular biologist Joshua Lederberg[7] who was awarded the Nobel Prize for his work that showed that microbes could "mate." He believed a germ-free world was hypothetically possible to create and would be something to think about regarding how to optimize human health in the future. But Koprowski rebutted that theory and argued that attempting to rid the world of microbes would disturb the delicate "truce" between microbes and humans "based upon the maintenance of ecological balance between man and the pathogenic bacteria."[8] He would later go on to suggest that rather than attempt to eradicate bacteria in the world, perhaps a better tactic would be to "implant man with a known concoction of living infective agents under controlled conditions rather than let him go germ-free into the world."[8] That is a strategy we now employ under the guise of products we call **probiotics.**

RISE OF THE BUBBLE BOY

For all the debate and logic that was pontificated on, the hubris of humankind led to a place, as it too often does, where the desire to answer questions about the possibility of germ-free human life outweighed the ethical concerns. The work by Reyniers and Trexler that led to the creation of germ-free animals eventually evolved into devices called isolators, used to isolate people (and their microbes) from those around them (and their microbes). Trexler, after separating from Reyniers for philosophical reasons, aimed to make these isolators available for clinical settings in order to protect both healthcare providers and patients from the spread of potentially deadly diseases such as Ebola.

That technology found its way into the hands of Ronald D. Barnes, a clinical scientist at the Institute of Child Health in London, who imagined that such isolators could allow for a germ-free isolation for humans—an answer for children who are born with severe immune dysfunction. Indeed, some of these children lived only a matter of months before succumbing to infection and death. With Trexler as his advisor, Barnes developed a hybrid isolator that would allow this hypothesis to be tested. A germ-free human would have to be raised and live out his or her life in isolation, just like any of the other germ-free species, and that was a point of contention among those involved. However, the ethical concerns became less of an issue when postulating the possible benefits of germ-free living for a child who would otherwise die if exposed to the microbes that are everywhere.

In 1968, the first successful germ-free human was born. However, it was found that the child did not have the immune dysfunction they thought he had, so he was only germ-free for a week. But in 1971, another child, David Vetter, was born germ-free under the care of Raphael Wilson, a gnotobiologist (someone who studies germ-free organisms) at the Texas Children's Hospital in Houston, Texas. David was born with a hereditary disease called severe combined immunodeficiency (SCID). His older brother had died of this condition soon after birth. So when given the choice, David's parents made the decision to be part of history, and David started his life as the world's first "bubble baby." David was even the subject of the 1976 movie *The Boy in the Plastic Bubble* starring John Travolta, and again in the 2001 movie *Bubble Boy* starring Jake Gyllenhaal (albeit in a more farcical take). However, despite the happy endings of both movies where the protagonist spontaneously recovers and leaves his bubble to start his romantically normal life, in reality, David Vetter died at the age of 12 due to complications following a bone marrow transplant from his sister.

One might wonder if such a venture would have been taken place if Barnes, Wilson, and Trexler had seen research on germ-free animals that was published well after David Vetter. That research would show that germ-free organisms can indeed live without microbes, but at a cost. Interestingly, some germ-free mice have been observed to even live longer than their microbe-laden counterparts; however, when the diets of conventionally born mice are restricted, that difference in lifespan seems to vanish.[9] So if scientists had stopped there, the case would have been settled—life without microbes may be the way to go if life span is not affected, and we could possibly avoid microbial-associated diseases that could prematurely reduce our lifespan such as the microbial culprit that causes hemorrhagic fever (Ebola, for instance). Having your cells explode and then bleeding to death isn't exactly a great way to go, and thus the argument for more bubble babies like David.

But observations did *not* stop there. They went much further and in the opposite direction. Despite the claims Cohendy made decades before, germ-free animals do not grow more quickly or larger than normal animals; in fact, they seemed to be smaller and weaker.[10,11] Germ-free animals have been observed to be functionally and structurally abnormal in quite a few of their bodily functions. They include dysfunction of the immune system, dysfunction of the digestive system, the inability to either make or absorb nutrients, irregular metabolism, and dysfunction of the nervous system.[12]

In the grand scheme of things, germ-free is *not* the way to go. Indeed, Pasteur has posthumously won the debate since it has become apparent that complex organisms require microbes in order to function properly. He also understood that it was a balance of making sure it was the *helpful* microbes that resided in the organism while the *harmful* ones were kept away. Regardless, the history of the pursuit of a germ-free existence has led us to know that our relationship with our microbes is not one from which we can simply walk away. And since we cannot escape this arranged marriage of sorts, it behooves us to do what it takes to live together in harmony.

Dr. Day: I saw a patient recently who came in double-masked and with a plastic visor over her face, wearing a trench coat and two pairs of latex gloves. She wiped down the exam chair before sitting down and kept her arms crossed the entire visit so as not to come in contact with any more surface than absolutely necessary. She mentioned that prior to COVID she was fine, but since the pandemic she had become completely obsessed with germs, and her entire day was focused on eliminating all germs from her skin and body. She was feeling helpless and despondent, and admitted it was ruining her life, but she feared for her life so she couldn't stop. She noted that she came into the office reluctantly because she had a breakout on her face, a stye on her left eye that would heal with medication but kept recurring once she stopped, and painful rashes on her hands that she knew were from overwashing. She didn't want to remove her mask or gloves to show me her concerns; instead, she brought out her phone and showed me photos. We discussed in detail that the breakout was due to overgrowth of microbes that don't normally live on the face; due to the face covering, microbes from her mouth would land on her skin and even along her eyelashes. The humidity would allow for overgrowth, and the friction from the mask would cause skin breakdown and lead to redness and further bacterial and yeast overgrowth, knocking out her skin's own natural microbiome and wreaking havoc. For all her efforts to be germ-free, she ended up with more germs—ones that were doing her far more harm than good.

AXES AND ALLIES

Despite the fact that the "anti-*culture* culture" is still somewhat pervasive in the West, a bit of awareness is beginning to emerge around the fact that living with microbes is inevitable. Despite the germ-free sentiments of yesteryear, more and more people are realizing that even if we cook our foods properly, even if we eat off the cleanest dishes using the cleanest silverware, even if we sterilize everything that goes into our mouths... even then, our guts are filled with massive amounts of microbes. Bacteria cover every surface we touch and float through the air we breathe, and so the skin is filled with massive amounts of microbes. That is why we will always be coated with microbes, inside and out. As we have alluded to, many of these microbes are essential for functioning—our allies, so to speak. However, there will always be some that can also make you sick.

Of all your organs, the gut contains arguably the most bacteria of anywhere both in and on your body. Your gut has a vast variety of bacteria, fungi, archaea, and viruses somewhere in the ballpark of 100 trillion organisms with a density in the colon estimated at 10^{11} to 10^{12} bacteria cells per milliliter. That's roughly the same number of bacteria in a milliliter of stool as there are stars in the entire Milky Way. Even more amazing is that a person weighing 150 pounds has about two and a half pounds of body weight comprised only of microbes. It is thus no surprise that dysbiosis in the gut microbiome has been associated with obesity, type II diabetes, inflammatory bowel disease, celiac disease, liver disease, cancers of the colon and liver, and neurologic conditions such as age-related macular degeneration, Alzheimer's, and Parkinson's diseases.

The same idea is true of the skin microbiome. There are an estimated 1 million bacteria for every square centimeter of our skin. That is likely a significant underestimate given the way skin microbiome samples have been captured. Regardless, like the gut, a dysbiosis of the skin micro-biome is associated with an array of disease states such as acne, psoriasis, atopic dermatitis, fungal infections, and so on. Having microbial allies in both the gut and the skin is essential to avoiding these issues.

The concept of being so saturated with microbes that it drives health and function may be somewhat disgusting to some, but it is a reality that most people can ultimately grasp and accept, albeit some more than others. We ultimately cannot prevent interaction of the surfaces of our bodies with microbes unless we live in a bubble—like David Vetter did. But what takes this cohabitation concept to the next level is that it is not just the outside surface of our bodies that enjoys cohabitation with microbes. Many other tissues of our bodies enjoy it as well, although not as extensively. For example, certain species of bacteria normally found on the skin (*Cutibacterium acnes*) have an interesting ability to live inside certain immune cells called macrophages and ride inside them throughout the entire body. It should be noted that these microbes can neither replicate inside these immune cells nor exit them.[13] However, they can have a significant effect on the way immune cells function. In fact, in biopsies of tissue, scientists isolated macrophages containing these microbes and found that the microbes actually have an immuno-suppressant effect on the surrounding cells.[14,15] Another example is when scientists looked in human blood plasma and found DNA from hundreds of new bacteria and virus strains previously known to be part of the human microbiome.[16]

While we continue to find more microbes in human tissues, you can rest assured that the number of microbes that live inside the body's tissues are magnitudes less than those that live in the skin and gut. The point is, however, that even in their small numbers, they can affect the human body either directly or indirectly. Much of the way microbes do this is by what is referred to as the gut-brain-skin (GBS) axis. That refers to a connection between these systems that allows the microbes of one system to affect the human tissues of another system.

For example, scientists have observed that the microbes in the gut may affect development of neurodegenerative diseases such as Parkinson's.[17] It isn't that the microbes cause the disease but that the presence of certain microbes—or more importantly the substances they produce when given certain diets—can communicate with the nervous system through the GBS axis and contribute to symptoms. Additionally, certain microbes can metabolize drugs that are meant to treat Parkinson's and can make them potentially less effective. When looking at the human gut in Parkinson's patients, it is clear that there is an altered microbiome there that is thought to contribute to an inflammatory state that aids in progression of the disease.[18] Whether the altered gut microbiota is due to a change in lifestyle due to the disease or a cause of the disease (or both) is still being studied, but regardless, there is an undeniable correlation between them.

However, more relevant to this book is the interconnection of the GBS in the pathology of skin disease. While it would make perfect sense that dysbiosis of the skin microbes leads to skin disease, there are also known correlations of gut microbes with skin diseases such as atopic dermatitis, psoriasis, rosacea, and even acne.[19] When we are looking at how to treat skin issues—whether disease, aging, or just looking your best—we should consider that it is not just the skin that needs to be addressed but the whole system, the **holobiont**. That includes the human, the microbes, and the environment from top to bottom and everywhere in between. They are all connected.

A WHOLE NEW MICROBIOME WORLD

It has been said that, like fingerprints, everyone has a unique microbiome. While this makes for a great headline, such a notion is still being investigated. Some parts of the microbiome are more universal than others, but we really need to determine if the parts that are not universal are unique over long periods of time or if they are simply due to everyday exposures that change as our locations or habits change. Many variables contribute to each person's microbiome from the time they are conceived to the time they take their last breath. Such variables include how long they were in the womb, the type of delivery by which they entered the world, whether they were bottle or breast fed, when they were weaned, what their diet is, what their body mass index is, how they exercise, what their lifestyle is like, what their cultural habits are, what medications they use, whether they have animals… the list goes on and on.

When we attempt to consider how a person might seek to curate their own "ideal" microbiomes, it behooves us to think about all the afore-mentioned variables and consider whether or not they are set or can be adjusted if or when needed. To begin to appreciate that, let's look at the earliest possible exposure to microbes—in the womb. Until very recently, it was thought that the womb where a fetus developed was a sterile environment and that the seeds for our body's microbiome came from our mother by way of the birth canal through which we enter the world. It was thought that microbes that live in the vaginal canal rub off as the baby squeezes through and engrafts to act as a microbial liaison when the baby leaves the sterile comfort of the womb and joins the ranks of a chronically contaminated environment. But what about those who are not born vaginally but by Caesarean section? They are not exposed to the same microbes in the same way. That does make a difference early on. There is an apparent shift in the microbiome of C-section born infants compared to those born vaginally. However, this apparent difference seems to normalize over time.[20] Interestingly, it has been observed that infants who are breast fed exclusively despite being born by C-section have microbes more similar to those of vaginally birthed infants.[21] So eventually, it all evens out. Factors other than mode of birth, including diet, actually play a role in the individual's microbiome composition.[22]

There is conflicting or even contradictory data from human studies suggesting associations of C-section birth and increased risk of a number of disorders, so it is not useful to assume that early differences in gut microbiomes lead to these issues.[23] Fortunately, babies born via Caesarean section are not quite as much at risk as once believed. A significant amount of recent research has shown that the womb is possibly not as sterile as we once thought and that we're likely exposed to a number of species of microbes while still growing within.[24,25] In fact, scientists have found in amniotic fluid two of the main species of skin microbes that stay with us throughout our lives—*C. acnes* and *S. epidermidis*.[22] Of course, they are in very small amounts, so scientists debate what that means. Some believe it is proof that our microbiomes begin to develop in the womb, while others believe it is no more than contamination of samples during the cited studies. While scientists are still figuring out the answers to questions such as how and when these microbes enter the uterus during gestation, where they come from, whether they are alive and replicating or dormant, and what function they play during development, we at least are seeing how soon in life our skin may be introduced to the microbes we'll then need to learn to live with.

When you consider the possibility that we are not born sterile, the idea does make sense. If we *were* sterile and born into a world teeming with microbes, our immune systems might go into shock or overreact during a critical period of life. After all, as we enter a world full of foreign microbes, we are bound to meet a new friend (or a million) in the very first minutes of life. Being exposed to microbes in the womb and early in life allows the body's developing immune system to slowly grow accustomed to the microbes it will need to learn to live with. Just as we can grow out of allergies when exposed to low levels of certain allergens, the adaptive immune system can learn when it's okay to leave certain microbes alone.

The skin microbiome we are born with keeps on colonizing as we grow and only begins to stabilize in adulthood. Does that mean we have a limited time to make sure we develop a healthy microbiome? Or do we have the ability to influence how our microbiome develops? These are the questions researchers are attempting to answer so in the future we can glean all the benefits of a symbiotic skin microbiome throughout our entire lives.

SKIN SPECIFICITY

Regardless of where our skin's microbiome comes from, it is relatively well established that there is a set number of known microbes that typically make up the constituents. In adults, the bacterial composition of skin is mostly dominated by the genera (plural for genus) *Cutibacterium, Corynebacteria,* and *Staphylococci.* Roughly 65% of skin microbes are made up of just those three genera. And when it gets down to the species level (species is a subclassification of genus), there are thousands of strains of bacteria that make up the skin's overall microbiome, yet most of the individual skin-related species make up less than 1% of the total microflora in any given skin site. There are major actors in the skin microbiome such as *C. acnes* and *S. epidermidis,* but the majority of strains found on the skin have what could be argued as minor roles.

Just because a type of bacteria is found in small numbers does not mean they are any less important or can't impart significant benefit—or harm. It's not necessarily only the presence of a microbe that creates a reaction, good or bad; it can also be the substances they produce. Since some microbes can make substances such as harmful endotoxins (what botox is derived from), a very tiny amount can have a large impact. However, sometimes the amount of microbes of a given species *is* important, especially when the molecules they secrete produce a protective benefit such as the copious antioxidants produced by *C. acnes* (discussed more in Chapter 3).

Of the literally thousands of bacteria species that can live on the skin, many of them (especially those that live on the surface) are transient in nature. In essence, they may be on your skin at any given moment because you touched something with those microbes already on it or have been sitting in a room where they are floating in the air and they simply land on your skin or you inhale them. Unless those transient microbes can find a hospitable surface of your body with the right kind of food (such as sweat or sebum) and the right location, pH, and so on, then they will eventually either die or shed off along with your dead skin cells. In other words, **just because a microbe finds its way onto your skin doesn't mean it will become part of your permanent skin microbiome.** When a given microbe strain ends up "taking" and becoming part of your long-term microbiome, it is called *engraftment*. As such, small changes in some of your skin's microbiome can happen over time. Think of it like a museum of microbes. Some exhibits are permanent, and others are temporary.

The change of those temporary "exhibits" over time is referred to as *temporal fluctuation* or *temporal variance*. Different skin sites have different levels of temporal fluctuation. Moist sites such as the armpit that are not directly exposed to objects we touch tend to have more stable bacterial communities over time. Drier and more exposed skin sites such as the palms seem to have a higher diversity of types of microbes and more changes to them over time. So the palms would have a higher temporal flux than the armpit.

Other terms used to describe the differences in microbiomes between skin sites is *alpha diversity* and *beta diversity*. Alpha diversity is the measure of how many types of species live in a given area on a person. Beta diversity is the measure of the differences of the microbiome composition when comparing different people. For example, a study showed that the inside of the arm, opposite the elbow, had the highest variance of microbiome species when comparing samples of different people—so it has a very high *beta diversity*. The same site on the body typically has very few unique species in that part of the microbiome, so it has a small *alpha diversity*.

Measures such as temporal flux and alpha and beta diversity can give us ways to assess the characteristics of any given microbiome in a particular area of the skin and how it functions. That is important so we can figure out how a microbe species might contribute to health or disease and how we might use that to our benefit. We could know how easy it would be to either get rid of a particular pathogenic strain or engraft a therapeutic strain that we might want in order to colonize the skin.

That said, once a microbiome is established, it is not typically easy to undo without long-term, consistent changes to the area where it lives. This was observed in studies where the popular acne treatment molecule benzoyl peroxide was used to reduce the overall number of bacteria on the face. The types and proportions of bacteria that were reduced at first eventually took up residence again when use of the medicine ended.[26] Although, there have been other studies that have shown that there are indeed changes in the diversity of the microbes post-treatment, how permanent any changes may be are inconclusive.[27] So while changing your microbiome for the better may be a fantastic idea for potential therapeutic applications, it is not often a simple task. It is possible, though, with long-term and consistent use of the right diets, products and habits. Some of these microbial modulation techniques will be discussed further in later chapters.

*Dr. Day: Alison, a 17-year-old junior in high school came in with her mom, complaining of worsening of her acne and with added irritation from all the products she was using. As I suspected, most of the products were aimed at erasing C. acnes and other bacteria from the skin. She was also regularly "cleaning" her skin with rubbing alcohol–soaked pads, thinking that would help clear her skin, but what she ended up with was irritated skin **and** pimples. She blamed the irritation on her "sensitive" skin. She felt that the only thing that helped her acne was going to the tanning salon since a tan helped hide her pimples and the redness and discoloration left behind from previous pimples.*

Her mom also added her concerns that her daughter's unhealthy diet of pizza and chocolate was causing the acne and she asked me to be sure to explain to her daughter how eating greasy foods makes the skin greasy and causes pimples. I had a lot of explaining to do to both the daughter, and the mom. The daughter had much relief when I said that grease from the pizza does not go directly to the skin and cause acne, unless she was directly rubbing the oil directly on her skin. I also had to explain to my patient that alcohol dries out and irritates the skin but doesn't have any effect on the bacteria she was trying to target, nor does it reach the base of the follicle where that bacteria lives. On top of that, going to the tanning salon was damaging and prematurely aging her skin, potentially ten times faster than from outdoor sun exposure and in the long run could also make her acne and the scarring worse. We discussed a personalized treatment protocol aimed at focusing on an antioxidant diet along with prescription and over the counter skin care products that helps support a healthy biome. She was excited to try it and was thrilled when not only her acne got better but she also felt better overall from the diet change that had long-lasting results.

In Dr. Day's clinical experience, her patients' onsets of acne were often correlated with times of stress such as students taking exams at school, changes in diet, and other life events. Some patients felt strongly that eating greasy foods correlated with their breakouts, but upon further investigation, we realized that there were other confounding variables such as staying up late studying for exams, changing a skin care routine around stressful times, and other factors that may have a greater effect than diet change alone. The distress acne causes can be devastating, and the scarring that too often goes with seemingly mild acne can be permanent. In her observation over more than twenty years of practice, Dr. Day has observed that acne scarring that seemed mild when patients were in their teens often looked severe as they aged and the skin increased laxity. That makes it even more important to understand the underlying causes of acne and to help prevent and treat it as early as possible to avoid the long-lasting emotional and physical effects it can cause.

SKIN DEEP

Much of the way information about the skin microbiome has been captured is by simply taking a sterile cotton swab, swiping the skin, and testing to see what grows from that swab sample. Many of us have had a physician swab somewhere on our bodies at one point in our lives so they can see if there is a potential microbe there that may be a problem for us. However, such a sampling technique is only good if what you are looking for is on the surface of what you are swabbing. Your skin's microbiome, however, is not only on the surface of the skin but also lies throughout the depths of your entire skin and beyond. So why are we drawing scientific conclusions when we are only sampling the surface? What's found beneath the surface may be even more important. That is also the case with gut microbiota. Many posit that the way we sample (via stool sample) may only reflect what *comes through* the GI tract, not necessarily what *lives in* the GI tract—a significant yet underappreciated distinction. More on this in **Chapter 8**.

Observations regarding incomplete sampling techniques and how that may lead us to incomplete conclusions can be allegorized by the poem "The Blind Man and the Elephant" by John Godfrey Saxe:

It was six men of Indostan
To learning much inclined,
Who went to see the Elephant
(Though all of them were blind),
That each by observation
Might satisfy his mind.

The first approached the Elephant,
And happening to fall
Against his broad and sturdy side,
At once began to bawl:
"God bless me! but the Elephant
Is nothing but a wall!"

The second feeling of the tusk,
Cried, "Ho, what have we here,
So very round and smooth and sharp?
To me 'tis mighty clear
This wonder of an Elephant
Is very like a spear!"

The third approached the animal,
And happening to take
The squirming trunk within his hands,
Thus boldly up and spake:
"I see," quoth he, "the Elephant
Is very like a snake!"

The fourth reached out his eager hand,
And felt about the knee
"What most this wondrous beast is like
Is mighty plain," quoth he;
"'Tis clear enough the Elephant
Is very like a tree!"

The fifth, who chanced to touch the ear,
Said: "E'en the blindest man
Can tell what this resembles most;
Deny the fact who can,
This marvel of an Elephant
Is very like a fan!"

The sixth no sooner had begun
About the beast to grope,
Than seizing on the swinging tail
That fell within his scope,
"I see," quoth he, "the Elephant
Is very like a rope!"

And so these men of Indostan
Disputed loud and long,
Each in his own opinion
Exceeding stiff and strong,
Though each was partly in the right,
And all were in the wrong!

Often scientists disagree and argue due to their perspectives. The data they produce may be incomplete for something as simple as sampling methods. However, in the field of skin microbiome, most scientists concede that this is indeed an issue that needs to be worked out. In the meantime, understanding the structure of skin and why a simple swab may not provide a complete picture of the skin microbiome is one way to avoid the "elephant in the room."

There are four main layers of the skin—stratum corneum, epidermis, dermis, and hypodermis. They are what most people consider when thinking about how topical products or medicines affect their skin. That is understandable because on the surface, your skin looks pretty flat. But when we look more closely, we see that skin is much more complicated. It isn't simply four main layers separated from each other like cake layers sandwiched with frosting between them. Instead, the skin's layers are interwoven and include secondary structures such as hair follicles, oil glands, and sweat glands that invaginate (fold back on each other to form a cavity) from one layer to another and transverse some or all the layers. This interconnectivity of layers is essential to skin function.

An example of this is the millions of pores that appear as small holes on the skin's surface. These are the entrances to hair follicles or sweat glands. While a layer of "dead" skin cells comprise the outermost layer of the skin, there is no stratum corneum inside the pores. However, the live epidermis below the surface stratum corneum flows right into and is the same as the cells that line each and every pore. The pore or hair follicle can extend from the surface of the skin all the way through the entire thickness of the skin's layers and into the fat or subcutaneous (deep) layers under the skin. There are many hundreds of thousands or millions of microbes in each pore. All those microbes, which are many more than what is on the surface, would not be represented correctly with a simple swab.

We must also consider how this distribution of microbes, given the anatomical feature of skin, would affect the interaction of the microbes with the human body. For many years, it was assumed that the gut had a surface area much larger than skin, but current thinking is that this isn't true. The gut's surface area is thought to be around 32 m², and the skin's is now estimated to be about the same. If so, that means the interface of the skin and its microbiome becomes one of if not *the* most significant of all our organs. And because the vast bulk of the skin's surface area—around a whopping 93%—is found within the hair follicles, then what lies beneath the surface carries that much more importance. So if we consider how much surface area of skin microbes have access to, we have to take into account not just the outermost surface but the surface area of all *5 million* or so hair follicles. That becomes even more pertinent when you consider that the skin is arguably the body's largest immune organ with dozens of immune cells surrounding each follicle. So the types of bacteria thriving within each hair follicle are very important to the health of our skin since they have the most access to our cells and immune system compared to the microbes that hang out on the surface.

As you can imagine, the environment of the hair follicle plays a huge role in determining which microbes might call it home. Follicles are filled with oils (or sebum) from the sebaceous glands, and these oils are what help seal our skin from the environment. The deeper into the follicle we go, the less direct access there is to air and oxygen. The bacteria that would do best in these conditions would be those that can thrive in our skin oils and don't require much, if any, oxygen. The bacteria that fit those qualifications are one of the major components of our skin microbiome, the *Cutibacterium acnes (C. acnes)* species of microbes. While Corneobacteria and Staphylococcus species such as *S. epidermidis* comprise much of our skin's surface microbiome, *C. acnes* is by far the most prevalent bacterial species of our skin microbiome. With the depths of our skin, it has the most access to our cells and immune system. Therefore, the way our *C. acnes* interact with our skin can have huge implications to our skin's health and beauty. **It's the one species that's so important that it gets its own chapter (Chapter 3).**

The Good, the Bad, and the Lethal

As you know by now, skin is the largest organ in the human body and provides protection from the environment. Given the state of our environment, it is inevitable that we will be covered in microbes either in the womb or moments before leaving it. As such, part of the function of our immune system is being able to determine which of these microbes are helpful, benign, or harmful. This function is essential since an imbalance or disruption of your body's healthy microbiome, called **dysbiosis**, can lead to health issues such as inflammatory diseases of the skin and gut, allergies, and certain cancers.

Unfortunately, these diseases are what most people immediately imagine when they think of microorganisms since some microorganisms can indeed do some pretty nasty things to us. Fortunately, not all microbes can grow on all parts of the skin, in part because the skin's surface is fairly dry. But the ones that *can* grow there but shouldn't, could leave your skin a mess—or worse. And it isn't just your immune system that functions to protect you from these unwanted microbes; it is your symbiotic microbes as well. A normal skin microbiome can help keep away all the nasty microbes almost as effectively as your immune system.

Not long ago, bacteria species such as *S. epidermidis* were labeled good, and *C. acnes* was labeled bad. After all, the species of acnes was named that since it was associated with acne. But many people who don't have any acne still have *C. acnes* as the most abundant bacteria species living in their skin all the time—while the supposedly good *S. epidermidis* is frighteningly the most frequent cause of hospital-derived sepsis, and interestingly also found in pores of those with acne more so than pores of those without acne.

What's become clear is that each species of bacteria might have several strains or subspecies, each with distinct physiological activities that might be considered good or bad, depending on when and where those activities take place. As we work on modulating the skin microbiome as a therapeutic way to address skin disease, knowing which bacterial **strains** (not just species) to target might be the key to successful treatment.

Since our sampling methods are still being refined so we can better understand where we want which microbes to be, it behooves us to respect our marriage of sorts to our microbes, as dysfunctional as it may sometimes seem. In the words of Louis Pasteur, "*Messieurs, c'est les microbes qui auront le dernier mot*" ("Gentlemen, it is the microbes who will have the last word.").

CHAPTER 3

SKIN'S MOST MISUNDERSTOOD MICROBE

There is nothing either good or bad,
but thinking makes it so.
—William Shakespeare, *Hamlet,* Act 2, Scene 2, 239–251

Shakespeare's *The Tragedy of Hamlet, Prince of Denmark*, typically referred to as simply *Hamlet*, has been considered one of the most influential and powerful tragedies written in the English language. For over four centuries, the tale of young, troubled Prince Hamlet has resonated with its audience through the exploration of universal themes of mental health, relationship dynamics and revenge. In this narrative, Hamlet is convinced of the validity of a spectral revelation that his father had been murdered by his uncle to usurp the crown. Talk about a life changing revelation! A large part as to why the tale of Hamlet has endured throughout the centuries is because many people can relate to the struggle of Hamlet as he deals with the upsetting and life-altering truth, wishing he simply did not such knowledge as it made his life much more uncomfortable, complicated, and, in his case, bloody. And while the revelation on the skin biome we are about to share with you in this chapter is hardly as dramatic – or bloody – as that of Hamlet's, it is indeed life altering. It was for us.

While Hamlet accepts the ghost's revelation as fact, one of the main narratives in the play is that he feels the need to force the truth to become evident to everyone else before he enacts his revenge on his uncle. While this book you're reading has nothing to do with any type of revenge plot, it is very much a means by which we are trying to make some relatively unknown (but pivotal) truths regarding the skin biome evident to everyone that we can. After all, knowledge is power, and we want everyone to have the power to be the healthiest and most beautiful version of themselves at every age. However, when we bring up the topic of skin bacteria, the most common responses are ones of disgust such as "eww, I don't want to hear about that" or "gross, I'd rather just not know" or "ignorance is bliss; let me stay ignorant." To that end, we chose the quote at the beginning of this chapter as we felt it conveys exactly the type of feeling that many go through when receiving such salient, albeit uncomfortable, knowledge. But we do not want the situation between you and your biomes to become a Shakespearian tragedy, and so it behooves us to get to know the key "actors" in our biome. But be forewarned, because in this next chapter some of you may find that a villain might become a hero, and likewise a friend might become a foe. So, prepare your mind, and in the words of Hamlet's father's ghost, we say to you, *"List, list, O, list!"*

Our revelation to you may seem provocative to some (at least at the time we are writing this), but this assertion is necessary to drive our discussion forward. The revelation is this: of all the microbes on the skin, there may be *one* species that is the most important for the health, balance, and symbiosis of the skin . . . *one* species that can affect our lives the most from birth to death . . . *one* bacterial species that, depending on the strain, can keep us looking younger for longer (we're guessing we now have your full attention). We assert that the most important species of the skin microbiome is the (unfairly) infamous *Cutibacterium acnes* (*C. acnes*). Cue the dramatic music!

To some of you, this declaration may be surprising or even shocking and unbelievable. You may feel incredulous, after all, for decades *C. acnes* has been regarded as the villain of the skin ecosystem, the "grey wolf" if you will. This species has been denigrated as a cause for diseases such as acne and the scarring and disfigurement that often goes with it. Many a product and procedure has been touted to have ability to diminish or even eradicate this species. Just like the grey wolf of Yellowstone in the early 20th century, "Death to the *C. acnes*" seems to linger as the dermatological battle cry.

To those who do find our assertion surprising, all we ask is that you suspend your disbelief for a moment and forget everything you *think* you know about *C. acnes*. Appropriate to the chapter's quote and like the play Hamlet puts on to expose his father's murderer, this chapter is going to flip the old thinking about *C. acnes*, acne treatment and skin health in general on its head. What we will cover here is a major fulcrum for why the Holobiont Philosophy is distinct from the way many of you may have cared for your skin until now. We will, of course, provide you with the rationale for why we are making such an assertion and why it is not simply our opinion but rather based on our own research and the research of many other thoughtful scientists.

So, let's dim the lights, raise the curtain, and enter the actors of the skin biome stage left.

FIRST LET'S MEET THE HERO OF THE STORY

Cutibacterium acnes, formerly known as *Propionibacterium acnes* or simply *P. acnes,* is a species of bacteria that is relatively slow-growing, doesn't really like oxygen (we call this an anaerobe) but can tolerate it if it has to, and loves to eat the oils of the skin as its primary food source, which makes its natural habitat and perfect home deep within the pores, aka follicles, of our skin. While many will know the species due to its association with the inflammatory skin issue known as acne vulgaris (for which the species was named), they may not know that every person on the face of the earth—yes, *everybody*—has *C. acnes* all over and inside their skin. That includes people with perfect skin who never had an acne blemish in all their lives. This species is, simply put, ubiquitous when it comes to the human skin. But at the current time, the most popular strategy is to attempt to eradicate *C. acnes* in order to help treat acne, a strategy still echoed by many skin health advocates and based on historical precedence. While this stance might be partially justified since some strains of *C. acnes* are associated with acne, it is only a small part of the overall picture and thus needs to be canceled as the status quo.

To understand the big picture, let's boil down some of what we know about the science behind this ubiquitous yet severely mischaracterized and misunderstood microbe. It is our hope that by the time you finish this chapter, you will stop thinking of *C. acnes* simply as an acne-causing villain to eliminate but rather as something we should strive to curate and cultivate.

NOT ALL *CUTIBACTERIA* ARE CREATED EQUAL

One of the biggest misconceptions when it comes to the microbiome in general is that all microbes in a given species are the same. That could not be farther from the truth. To demonstrate this point, let's consider several ingredients currently found in skin care products with claims of being "probiotic" (this list is by no means exhaustive).

- *Bifida* Ferment Lysate

- *Lactococcus* Lysate Ferment

- *Lactobacillus*

- Lactic acid bacteria

If we compare two products with, say, *Lactobacillus*, it may be assumed that both products contain the same probiotic ingredient. However, *Lactobacillus* is a genus, a larger group of organisms that many species fall under. That means there are many species that fall under the umbrella of this group of bacteria. In fact, there are at least 100 species of *Lactobacilli*.

So should you consider *Lactobacillus acidophilus* the same as *Lactobacillus salivarius?*

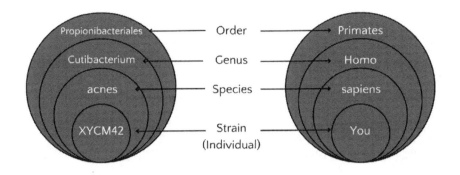

Don't feel badly if you don't know the answer to that. Most people don't know the difference. The ignorance of the general public of this matter is reasonable, but nevertheless something that less scrupulous supplement companies may take advantage of. Reality is, while the two distinct species of microbes in the same genus will have some similarities since they *are* related, they will also have many significant differences. After all, scientists don't simply assign different species designations for the heck of it. They do so because there are distinct differences in the species' genetics, differences in what they secrete, and differences in how they function overall. To assume that all *Lactobacilli* are the same can be likened to assuming that a coyote (*Canis latrans*), a jackal (*Canis aureus*), and a wolf (*Canis lupus*) are all the same as they are all are under the genus, *Canis*. Yes, they have similarities, but there is a distinct reason why they have different names.

While this example is about differences among microbes in the same genus, let's now consider differences in microbes of the same species since they should be even more closely related than those in a whole genus. To keep the same example of the genus *Canis*, let's look at a subspecies within the species *Canis lupus*—the grey wolf (our friend from Yellowstone National Park discussed in Chapter 1). Under this subspecies are sub-subspecies (or strain in microbial talk)—the Eurasian wolf (*Canis lupus*

lupus) and the well-known *Canis lupus familiaris,* or simply *Canis familiaris,* otherwise known as man's best friend - the dog. The wolf and the dog the same species but are very different animals. One will lick you as a form of affection, and the other one would rather kill you…and your dog.

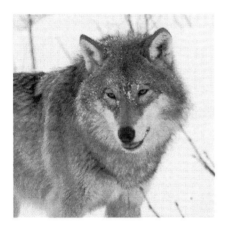

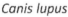

Canis lupus

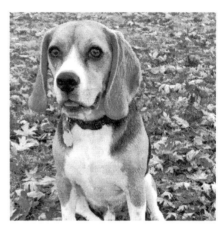

Canis familiaris

This analogy translates directly to the microbiome. As we learn more and more about the interaction of the microbiome with our human cells, we are starting to realize that the benefits we observe when using probiotic bacteria is not universal but very specific to the strain. Even within the same species of microbe, there can be significant differences, just like those between a wolf and a beagle. These differences between microbes in the same species can range from quite extreme to inconsequential. However, they can be the difference between life and death with regard to how they affect us as humans. When we hear about strains of bacteria that become antibiotic-resistant, we are comparing microbes in the same species, but one is antibiotic-resistant, and the other is not. That is a significant and concerning difference.

This is the case with the species *C. acnes.* This species is ubiquitous, but what we have quite recently learned is that there are important, distinct groupings of characteristics that can be found in many of the hundreds (if not thousands) of strains of *C. acnes*. The differences between the strains of *C. acnes* have been found to be so significant that scientists have recently revised the naming convention for the following few major groupings of strains within the *C. acnes* species by what we refer to as phylotypes (groups of strains that have a common genetic association).

- phylotype 1 – *C. acnes* subspecies *acnes* – (strains most associated with disease)

- phylotype 2 – *C. acnes* subspecies *defendens* – (strains most associated with health)

- phylotype 3 – *C. acnes* subspecies *elongatum*

There are quite a few details about what makes these groupings distinct, but we will not get into them for the sake of simplicity. We do want to give you a few key nuggets about why all *C. acnes* are not the same.

CORRELATION, CAUSATION, AND CUTIBACTERIA

As mentioned, *C. acnes* has long been implicated as *the* primary cause for acne. While it must be conceded that there are strains of *C. acnes* that have a very strong association with acne, it simply cannot be dismissed that there are also those that have almost no association with acne. Additionally, as we are about to examine, there are some strains that may even be considered symbiotic. So should we really be trying to kill them all?

While there are some associations of specific subspecies of *C. acnes* with either health or disease, it is not simply the presence of any single strain of *C. acnes* that is *the* cause of disease. There is evidence of correlations of certain strains to those who have acne, but it is much harder to prove causation, that those strains directly cause the disease. This is apparent when comparing samples of acne sufferers' microbiomes with those of healthy individuals. While studies have shown that certain strains are exclusive to the skin of those who have acne, usually there is a mix of several strains that inhabit all people's skin.[1] Additionally, for all the talk about *C. acnes* causing acne, little is said about the fact that multiple studies have shown that acneic skin actually has **less** *C. acnes* and more microbial diversity, including an increase in the (sometimes) commensal *Staphylococcus epidermidis*, especially in hair follicles.[23] Those with perfectly clear skin can have the same strains as those who have acne and yet may hardly ever see a blemish. That is because it is not just the presence of any particular strain(s) of *C. acnes* but also just as important (if not more important) is what *other* microbes are involved and the way your skin and immune system respond to the presence of those strains, as well as any substances they may produce.

A study on this idea sought to see how immune cells from various people may react differently to the same *C. acnes* strain.[3] In the study, researchers took immune cells from both healthy and acne individuals and treated them with the same strain of *C. acnes*. What was observed was that the immune cells of both groups had an increase in inflammatory signals; however, the acne patients' cells were not able to produce enough anti-inflammatory substances, to counteract this upregulation of inflammatory genes. Simply put, the cells of the people with acne were more predisposed to being inflamed. That is in part why two people can have the same microbes on their skin but only one may have acne while the other does not.

Even though the presence of any strain does not solely dictate health or disease, the strains do matter. It has been observed that the strain of *C. acnes* that is present may actually influence your immune system to be either more prone to either inflammation or quiescence.[4] Even more, a health-associated strain of *C. acnes* can influence your immune system to attack the disease-associated *C. acnes*.[5] So while a given strain of *C. acnes* may contribute to acne, other *C. acnes* strains can actually help train your immune system to prevent acne. It could be that some strains of *C. acnes* may be just as protective to your skin as the pathogenic strains are detrimental.

Using our analogy again, in the past we considered all the wolf species (or our *C. acnes*) "bad." Now when we look at the strain level, we see that while the grey wolf (or our *C. acnes* subspecies *acnes*) might cause a bit of trouble if left unchecked, the beagles (or our *C. acnes* subspecies *defendens*) help police them. Most places may have a mix of grey wolves, beagles, and any number of other animals, but it seems that too many grey wolves can cause an imbalance in the ecosystem. While a beagle might not be a match for a grey wolf in a fight, the beagle can win overall by signaling to its human master (or in our analogy, the immune system) the wolf's presence, and the master can remedy the situation with a shotgun. But should we completely eradicate the grey wolf (*C. acnes acnes*)? Could they serve another purpose that we just don't currently understand? Perhaps that is where our analogy breaks down, or perhaps we need to take a page from the Yellowstone story and remember that it is all about balance.

NOTING THE DIFFERENCES

What are some of the key differences between the phylotypes of *C. acnes* strains that makes them more or less prone to be associated with disease? Many of the differences can be seen by comparing the genetic information of each strain. Some *C. acnes* strains can have more genes than other strains, and the way the genes are expressed can also be quite different. But why? To understand why such genetic differences exist within strains of the same species of bacteria, we must know a little microbiology 101.

Bacteria typically only have one chromosome made up of a closed loop of DNA.

Human DNA

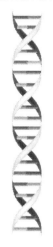
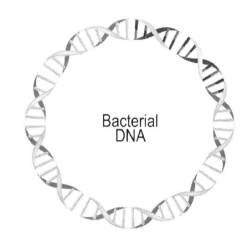

Bacterial
DNA

Some have a smaller loop called a plasmid. However, there are a few ways bacteria can receive new genetic information. One way is by a sort of microbial sexual reproduction called bacterial conjugation where a donor cell sends a copy (sometimes a full copy and sometimes a partial one) of its plasmid to a recipient cell. If that happens, the recipient cell now has new genetic material that can potentially be incorporated into its permanent genetic code. Another way is through a process called transformation where the DNA of a dead bacterium can be ingested into a live bacterium and incorporated into its own chromosome. A final way is by a process called transduction where a phage (a bacteria-specific virus) attaches to a bacterium and injects its genetic information into the cell, which then can sometimes incorporate that DNA if it doesn't cause it to explode instead. Regardless of the way it happens, a bacterium can be "offered" new genetic code that can then be placed into its own chromosome and result in some sort of change to the overall function and metabolism of the organism and its offspring.

A prime example of this is one way antibiotic-resistant genes can be transferred from pathogenic microbes and are propagated. Another is the disruption of normal gene regulation in other systems such as causing an upregulation (producing more) or downregulation (producing less) of a particular gene's products. That can result in a bacterium secreting or not secreting substances that might be harmful to the human host when it shouldn't and when it normally wouldn't. That can be observed among the various strains of *C. acnes*. If you look at those strains, as well as the things they have in their DNA and what they secrete, you can see distinct differences. One example of these differences is a series of five genes called CAMP genes that all *C. acnes* have, whether their phenotype is associated with pathogenicity or health.[6] However, the *C. acnes* that tend to be associated with disease seem to upregulate the gene for CAMP2, 3 and 5 and downregulate the gene for CAMP1. The opposite is true for *C. acnes* strains that are associated with healthy skin. These are the same genes in the same species (albeit different strains) of bacteria, yet they are functioning very differently, which changes how they affect their human hosts.

There is also an argument that the *C. acnes* associated with healthy skin is a purer form of the *C. acnes* species. That means it's possible that all *C. acnes* started out the same, and then by the addition of genes (by the above three methods), strains slowly diverged into those that functioned differently due to the changes in the genetic code. But why would some *C. acnes* stay pure while others went to the dark side? Well, it is not known exactly, but one clue is in a special genetic element called CRISPR. This element is like a primordial immune system specifically found in some bacteria that keep foreign DNA out. Many of the protective *C. acnes* that are associated with health have a working CRISPR element, while many of the pathogenic *C. acnes* associated with disease do not. Thus we should consider the various groupings of *C. acnes* as distinct, almost separate.

IMPLICATIONS OF DIVERSITY

One of the current mantras that can be found in both the skin care and gut health arenas is that more diversity in the kinds of microbes in the microbiome equals a healthier microbiome. While this can be true in some areas of the body, it is not necessarily a universal rule when it comes to all the skin biomes. There are also times when healthy skin is associated with *less* diversity. That might come across at first blush as contradictory and confusing, but when we remember that like most ecosystems the skin is not homogenous in nature, it starts to make more sense. Not only are there stark differences to the variable areas of the skin (dry torso, wet underarms, oily face, etc.) but there are also stark differences between what lives on the oxygen-rich surface and what lies within the oily, oxygen-poor hair follicle or pore. An example of when skin microbiota diversity has been associated with skin health is what some studies have found when comparing relatively healthy-skinned people to those with atopic dermatitis. The disease is correlated to areas of skin where there is less diversity and a higher than typical prevalence of *Staphylococcus aureus* and interestingly a dearth of *C. acnes*. A contrast to that is in research from Dr. Li's lab and corroborated by other labs that more diversity (and less *C. acnes*) is found in those who have acne. You can now see the point that diversity does not always equal a healthy microbiome, especially when it comes to the skin and *C. acnes*.

CUTIBACTERIA AND COSMESIS

As we've already discussed, the interplay between our human cells and the skin microbiome's most prevalent species, *C. acnes*, is nuanced and somewhat complicated. How we get along with this species depends on us (our genetics, the environment we provide) and them (the particular strain, how it reacts to the environment we provide). It depends on the skin biome as a whole, and there is a give and take by each—a bit of a dance, if you will. When you boil it all down, the way in which *C. acnes* strains can significantly affect overall skin health and beauty is by their interaction with human cells via the substances they secrete.

1. **Human/*C. acnes* cell interaction.** Since it was thought for a long time that *C. acnes* was the cause of acne, it was assumed that it also caused the hallmark inflammation that acne sufferers know all too well. This

assumption was not all together wrong since there was indeed a good portion of *C. acnes* subspecies *acnes* that contributed to inflammation. Many scientific studies used strains of *C. acnes* subspecies *acnes* to instigate inflammation so some new pharmaceutical or nutraceutical ingredient could be tested to see how it might stop the inflammation caused by these strains (or simply kill the strains outright). However, we now know that certain strains do not necessarily instigate inflammation in human cells.

Dr. Hitchcock: When I started my lab, Xycrobe Therapeutics, in San Diego, my main goal was to find a strain of microbe in the skin microbiome that would act as a perfect vehicle to deliver therapeutics into the skin. When we stumbled across a strain of C. acnes defendens from a volunteer's skin swab, we thought it might be a great candidate since it had all the correct markers that made us think it would be commensal (harmless) and therefore a good vehicle. However, when we started testing the strain with human skin cells, human skin explants, and human immune cells, we were blown away that not only did the C. acnes strain not cause any inflammation signaling to occur in any of the models, but it stopped inflammation even when we attempted to cause it. That was an aha moment because it told us that certain strains of C. acnes may not simply be commensal but may even be somewhat symbiotic in nature.

As mentioned earlier, research has shown that the strain of *C. acnes* is very important since protective *C. acnes* strains can serve to train certain immune cells to become either inflammatory or quiescent.[7] While a particular strain may not directly cause skin disease or acceleration of aging via inflammation, it can definitely encourage those things. The good news is that if the current research is correct, then as long as we foster a good environment for our skin microbiota (i.e., not overwashing or applying harsh topicals), the protective strains will train the immune system to slowly but systematically target the pathogenic strains until some sort of balance is achieved. And remember that the protective strains such as *C. acnes defendens* tend to have CRISPR elements to protect them against phage attack. The pathogenic strains often do not. This is also good news for our skin. But the bad news is that the pathogenic strains tend to be more robust and fast growing than the protective strains. So if we abuse our microbiomes or try to sterilize our skin, it is the pathogenic strains that very well might get the upper hand. But if we take care of the skin microbiome's environment, chances are that eventually good will prevail.

2. **The substances *C. acnes* secrete (microbioforming).** There are several substances that *C. acnes* produces during its metabolic process. Some are critical to your health and the beauty of your skin. These substances help mold the skin environment to be conducive to the curation of the very best skin microbiome, leading to healthy and radiant skin. The continuous contribution of metabolites of the *C. acnes* on our skin is reminiscent of what occurs in the process of "terraforming" in science fiction literature. That is when an inhospitable planet is transformed by some sort of technological means to make it resemble earth so it can support human life. In a way, *C. acnes* does the same thing to make the skin hospitable for a symbiotic microbiome. Dr. Hitchcock thus likes to combine the words *microbiome* and *terraforming* to come up with the term *microbioforming*. While Dr. Hitchcock uses this term tongue in cheek, it does help describe how protective strains of *C. acnes* participate in the formation and upkeep of an optimal skin environment.

The first substance *C. acnes* produces that we want to highlight is propionic acid (PA). *C. acnes* makes this substance in copious amounts, which is why they were originally under the genus *Propionibacterium*. Propionic acid is one of the skin's healthy short chain fatty acids (SCFA) that you should covet for your skin. This molecule is created by *C. acnes* through its metabolism of your skin oil secretions. It is quite an unsung hero when it comes to microbioforming, skin health, and beauty. What does propionic acid do for the biome?

- **Targets antimicrobials.** PA has been shown to actively suppress the growth of *Staphylococcus aureus*, including MRSA, and to exhibit broad-spectrum antimicrobial activity against *Escherichia coli* and *Candida albicans* as well.

- **Lowers skin pH.** While commensals and symbiotes love the low pH of our skin, the pathogens (like *S. aureus*) don't particularly like low pH.

- **Inhibits *Staph* biofilm formation.** Formation of *Staphylococcus* biofilms can contribute to skin disease.

- **Inhibits tyrosinase.** PA has been shown to influence the production of pigment by inhibiting tyrosinase, just like vitamin C.

- **Exfoliates.** Helps keep the turnover of skin cells smooth.

- **Serves as an antioxidant.** We will cover this next.

The second substances that *C. acnes* produces in copious amounts are antioxidants, which are critical to keeping free radicals and oxidative stress (reactive molecules that significantly contribute to aging, inflammation, and cancer) to a minimum. It is a huge boon for us that the most prevalent microbe that lives not only on but also deep inside the skin secretes a huge amount of not one but multiple types of antioxidants. One of them is the salt form of PA that we already discussed. Another is a molecule that is unique to the *C. acnes* species, called RoxP. This antioxidant is stable and has been shown to be as powerful as vitamin C. However, an advantage over vitamin C is that RoxP is produced on your skin already if you have a healthy and balanced microbiome (with lots of protective *C. acnes*) in large amounts at all hours of the day. All you have to do is foster it. Research has shown that RoxP contributes to the viability of immune cells and skin cells exposed to free radical stress.

Reductions in *C. acnes* (and thus RoxP) have been associated with oxidative diseases such as some forms of skin cancer.[8] In addition to RoxP, scientists in Dr. Hitchcock's lab have identified at least one other small molecule in the ferment of protective *C. acnes* strains that is just as potent as RoxP. The identity of this mystery antioxidant is yet to be determined; however, it contributes to the case that having copious amounts of protective *C. acnes* strains on your skin is a good thing.

The next substance we want to add to this list of protective *C. acnes* offerings is bacteriocins. An example is cutimycin, an antibiotic produced specifically by *C. acnes* and targeted at *Staphylococcus* species, including both *S. aureus* and *S. epidermidis*. That is key since it helps keep *S. epidermidis* isolated to the surface where they can be commensal and away from the follicles where they can possibly throw the biome out of whack. There are at least two other bacteriocins found in the different types of *C. acnes*, each with its own specificity to what it either kills or inhibits. However, most of the time it related to keeping *Staphylococcus* species at bay and out of the follicles.

Next are anti-inflammatory molecules. They are a bit more elusive as to what they are and how they act, but what we know is that something protective *C. acnes* strains secrete can act to lower inflammation in the skin. In works published by Dr. Hitchcock's lab in 2022, topical application of a protective strain of *C. acnes* showed a reduction of inflammatory gene signals in both skin models as well as a clinical reduction in symptoms of inflammation after clinical use.[9]

Finally, we want to discuss the molecules that some *C. acnes* strains secrete that may not be so great. But fortunately, the amounts secreted by the protective strains tend to be little to none. They are called porphyrins, a group of molecules that are part of the biosynthesis of essential components of living organisms such as heme and chlorophyll. Porphyrins secreted by *C. acnes* can be pro-inflammatory when secreted at high levels since they interact with ultraviolet rays (UV) from the sun and release free radicals into the skin. When high levels of porphyrins are found (via woods lamp) on the skin, it tends to be correlated with inflammatory skin issues, primarily acne vulgaris. The good news is that scientists have shown that the protective strains of *C. acnes* secrete *significantly* less (almost none in comparison) porphyrins than their pathogenic counterparts.[10,11] In addition, studies have shown that the healthy *C. acnes'* low level of porphyrin secretion is pretty consistent where the pathogenic *C. acnes* tends to increase porphyrin production when given certain food sources such as meat and dairy that contain high levels of vitamin B12). That may be why some people tend to break out with acne when they ingest certain foods while others never have any problems.

LEARNING TO LOVE YOUR CUTIBACTERIA

So far, we have laid out the argument for our premise that *C. acnes* is the most important microbe on and in your skin. However, we do not claim that it is the *only* important skin microbe since any microbe that contributes to benefits or detriments for the skin is also very important. We have shown that *C. acnes* is ubiquitous among the human population and that the benefits it brings to the skin are on par with the best skin care ingredients. The caveat is that while the good forms of *C. acnes* should be protected and fostered, the bad strains of *C. acnes* are just as important in the sense that if they manifest disease, it can affect your quality of life. While in our chapter quote Shakespeare's Prince Hamlet may have preached that ignorance is bliss, now that you are armed with this information, you can choose to use it to help you achieve better balance in your biome.

The great news is that if you develop habits that foster the right environment for our protective *C. acnes* to grow and flourish, then eventually your biome can find a way to bring your skin into balance. But modern-day skin care routines don't make it easy since so much of it is often specifically designed to destroy *C. acnes*. Our advice is to embrace the oils of your skin, be picky about the cleansers you use, and watch when and how often you use them since they can lead to oil (and subsequently *C. acnes*) dysregulation. You only need to wash off the surface dirt. Anything more will strip your skin biome and cause it to be off balance. The oils of your skin are utopia for your protective *C. acnes* that naturally provide copious and consistent amounts of SCFA, antioxidants, anti-inflammatories, and more. Who knows what we will discover next? There must be a reason why anecdotally those with oily skin tend to age better. So when you are putting together your biomecare regimen (we will help with this in Chapter 7), keep in mind your *C. acnes* and the environment they love. Then seek to curate your *C. acnes* since now more than any time in history, new innovations are coming into the market that can help you achieve symbiosis with your microbes. Having the right *C. acnes* is a big part of the Holobiont Philosophy that will help your skin avoid tragedy—Shakespearean or otherwise.

PART II
RETHINKING THE BIOME

CHAPTER 4

FEAR AND LOATHING IN LAS BIOME

Do the best you can until you know better.
Then when you know better, do better.
—Maya Angelou

We expect there to be some skepticism around the topic of the last chapter. It does flip roughly sixty years of medical tradition on its head to think that *C. acnes* is not the microbial devil incarnate it has been made out to be, but that it may actually be a guardian angel when it comes to skin health. We hope we were able to convey to you that the most current research has provided information proving that something we thought was straightforward and immutable is more complicated than we initially thought, and now we need to change our strategies of how we care for the skin biome. We have gone from the previous standard of care which declares "all *C. acnes* bacteria *cause* disease and must be eradicated to a more appropriately balanced declaration that "some *C. acnes* strains are essential for proper skin health and some strains may *contribute* to disease."

However, we should not let our collective scientific and medical ego get in the way of learning from our past to do better for ourselves in the future. After all, for a long time in human history microbes were a huge unknown. Even when they were eventually discovered, they were not well understood (and still not completely so). As we know, humans have a tendency to fear the unknown, villainize the misunderstood, and act irrationally toward both those things. Thus, it is natural for those who have practiced *microbial genocide* as the standard of care for decades to resist the change of mindset to **microbial curation**. Per this chapter's quote by Maya Angelou, we did our best with what we knew. However, we now know more…we know better, and therefore can do better.

Despite human tendencies to fear the unknown and resist change, reflecting on history gives us some perspective and allows us to step back and take a look at the potential evolution of our medical and sanitary practices in light of other historical advances in knowledge. This is important to do at this juncture in history, as we are in a sort of renaissance period when it comes to microbiome science, especially of the skin. One of the oldest examples took place in most pre-modern societies when religious superstitions ruled without scrutiny. One example is the Aztec Empire of the fourteenth to sixteenth centuries. During that time the Mexica people in what is now Mexico believed strongly that it was in the best interest of all people to have a standardized practice of human sacrifice. It was thought that without human sacrifice "the sun would cease to rise and the world would end."[1] And of course, as is the case with martyrdom in most religions, the sacrificial victims would then earn a "special, honored place in the afterlife."[2] They were convinced that this was the reality of this world and that only human sacrifice "would feed the gods and ensure the continued existence of the world." Not only was this a standard routine but the victim's remains were expertly processed and enshrined in sophisticated structures and used as ceremonious garb. Today we might consider this irrational because we know that the sun rises and sets due to the spinning of the earth and that there is nothing that any person needs to do to perpetuate this natural phenomenon. We know more now, and therefore we don't find it necessary to sacrifice our neighbors.

Another less dramatic example that is more medically relevant is bloodletting, the practice of removing blood from a person's veins for alleged therapeutic reasons. Until the late nineteenth century, this practice was accepted as the standard of care for many ailments with the thought pattern described by the notable Hippocrates (~460–370 BC) that illness was caused by an imbalance of the four humors (blood, phlegm, black bile, yellow bile). To relieve the patient of illness, they had to be relieved of the imbalanced humor. When Galen of Pergamum (129–200 AD) declared blood as the most dominant humor, the practice of bloodletting took a prominent place in medicine for about the next 2,000 years.[3] However, despite how popular the practice was in medicine, and how long it persisted, only a few examples of the practice is used in medicine today (for more scientific reasons we would hope).[4] We know more now and therefore we have stopped draining our patients of their blood. For thousands of years, practices such as human sacrifices and bloodletting were performed routinely, standardized, and thought to be legitimate until we learned we were doing things that were quite bad and unnecessary for those whom these practices were acted out upon and did nothing that was legitimately beneficial for the rest of society.

As we have already discussed, due to some scientific misconceptions of the recent past, many take an extreme approach to cleanliness by attempting to sanitize their surroundings and even their own bodies. If we lived in a relatively sterile world, that would be a strategically wise thing to do. But we do *not* live in a sterile world. As we have seen, nearly every nook and cranny of the world is teeming with microbes. Some can live in our bodies, but many cannot. Some produce toxic substances, and many do not. Some even produce substances that can do miraculous things! That has been observed countless times, one of the most notable being the observation by Alexander Fleming in 1928 that a culture dish of *Staphylococcus* bacteria that he accidentally left uncovered was contaminated by a certain *other* microbe, a fungus called *Penicillium notatum*. He observed that wherever the fungus grew on the dish, there were zones surrounding it where the bacteria could not grow. Fleming had stumbled upon the fact that many microbes produce substances that are actually antimicrobial—how is that for irony? For the sake of clarity, microbes produce substances that are antimicrobial against microbes *other* than themselves, usually very select microbes. In this case, Fleming had observed that this *Penicillium* fungus could indeed kill types of *Staph-*

ylococcus bacteria. Yes, Fleming had discovered the antibiotic penicillin which changed the world of medicine, and he was aptly awarded the Nobel Prize in Physiology/Medicine in 1945, along with Howard Florey and Ernst Chain for bringing the first mass produced antibiotic to the world.

As an interesting side note, Dr. Day's uncle, Dr. Atta Bakshandeh, was influential in creating a fat-soluble version of penicillin in the 1950s that extended its shelf life and enabled it to be exported throughout the world. He and Dr. Day's father instilled in her the value and love of research and medicine.

As amazing as Fleming's discovery was, it's important to note that selectable antimicrobial substances derived from certain microbes had been around and used for millennia. Although it wasn't known that microbes were involved in causing infections, ancient civilizations used various fungi, plant extracts, and even honey to treat most skin ailments. While they didn't understand why wrapping a wound with moldy bread or a compress soaked in honey might help, modern science has uncovered that even the tiniest of creatures (i.e., bacteria) can secrete multiple bioactive substances that work in concert to protect themselves and, in turn, protect their hosts. As we saw in Chapter 2, we are now discovering how the protective microbes that call our bodies home also secrete a myriad of bioactives, including such antimicrobial substances, many that are essential to the health and beauty of our skin.

When it comes to diseases associated with pathogenic microbes, even the experts still debate whether it's the microbes that cause the disease or the disease state itself that creates an environment that fosters these microbes—or maybe a bit of both. A growing body of evidence links certain skin diseases to specific types of microbes. So as there is indeed a link between microbiome dysbiosis and skin disease, we should realize that a literal war is constantly being fought in our skin, but it isn't as simple as humans versus microbes. Sometimes microbes attack humans; sometimes they don't. Sometimes the human cells attack the microbes, and sometimes they don't. And sometimes microbes turn on other microbes, and sometimes they don't. We have begun to see how complex the interaction of the human body with its microbiomes is, and that how disease manifests via this interaction is anything but simple. The real question is this: What does this mean for how we treat diseases and how we might prevent them in the first place? Now that science is showing us a more complex story that underlies the undeniable link between our health and our microbiomes, is it wise to continue the traditional ways of addressing skin issues associated with microbes? Perhaps it is time to explore what it might mean to do better now that we know better.

Causation versus Correlation

One of the first things taught in introductory statistics textbooks is that correlation is not causation. It is also one of the first things forgotten.
—Thomas Sowell

The concept of causation versus correlation—whether a microbe causes the disease or if the microbe just happens to be there because of the disease—is of significant importance to the skin biome. For decades, certain microbes have been blamed for causing skin issues, and thus clinicians make decisions on how to treat based on the assumption that it is a certain microbe that *causes* the issue. What does causation versus correlation mean in context of the skin biome?

- **Correlation:** The association between two items or variables

- **Positive correlation.** An increase in one item or variable directly affects an increase in another item or variable, and vice versa (e.g., temperature goes up; ice cream sales go up).

- **Negative correlation.** An increase in a variable, leads to a decrease in another variable (e.g., if I increase my exercise, I decrease my weight).

- **No correlation.** The two variables do not have any relationship to each other (e.g., coffee consumption vs. intelligence).

Causation: When two variables have a cause-and-effect relationship with one another (e.g., driving while drunk causes more car accidents)

It is quite common to see correlation and causation at the same time. That is the case for a couple of our previous examples. In the summer months, for example, the temperature rises, which causes people to seek out cooling activities such as eating ice cream. The correlation is also causative in nature. Likewise, by exercising you are causing your body to lose fat and weight. This correlation is also causative. However, it should be noted that correlation *does not imply* causation. That is called the false cause fallacy, or wrongly assuming that one thing causes another simply because they have a relationship of some kind. An example is ice cream sales versus shark attacks. If you look at a trend of ice cream sales and shark attacks, you will notice that they tend to have a positive correlation —when one goes up or down, often the other one does too. But this is not because ice cream sales cause shark attacks, or vice versa. It is because ice cream sales tend to rise in the summer months as do the occurrence of shark attacks. However, there is not a causative link between them.

The false cause fallacy is something that should always be considered when discussing the skin microbiome and its association with skin disease. Quite a bit of research shows a very strong correlation of certain species of microbes to skin disease. A couple of prime examples of this are the associations of *C. acnes* with acne or *Staphylococcus aureus* with atopic dermatitis. But are these associations simply correlative, or are they causative? Let's discuss some of these associations of microbes with disease states and see if our knowledge of how they are implicated in the disease can help determine a better way to treat the issue. Note that we won't discuss *all* the diseases associated with microbes since that would be a very long chapter.

AGING SKIN

When we look in the mirror and see signs of aging, like wrinkles, sun (age) spots, broken blood vessels or blotchy skin, and gray hair, we are hard-wired to see that as a sign of trouble and to want to make it better since older age is generally associated with loss of fertility and functional decline. However, one of the shared experiences we all face during our lives is aging. The fact is that we all age, and our skin gives off one of the most visible telltale signs of our age. While seeing the signs of aging is not necessarily enjoyable, we can learn to see beauty in someone who has aged well and even to see it as a greater beauty than that of youth since it comes with a life that has been lived, and often a life of purpose.

We can also take steps to help our skin and our bodies age healthier and even undo some of the damage that has already occurred. Stop and think about it. If we look healthy, then we will look beautiful and appropriate at any age. Brilliant scientists are working on possible ways to slow down and even reverse the biology of human aging, but we aren't quite there yet. The most reliable way to prevent premature aging is by taking care of our skin—by using sunscreens, eating a proper diet, exercising regularly, getting enough sleep, taking care of our microbiome, and not over washing. In Chapters 7 and 8, we will cover some of the Biomecare strategies to keep skin age appropriately healthy.

When it comes to skin, there is a huge desire for anti-aging properties in topical products. There are some ingredients that can impact skin aging; however, the term *anti-aging* at face value can be a bit deceptive. Consumers are led to think of this term as a claim to turn back the clock, which is not a realistic claim for most products. Most aesthetic products simply mask the signs of aging. We will explain how the skin biome as a whole play into aging and then show you how to begin to slow down or even reverse the skin aging process. Since the skin biome consists of both our human skin cells and our skin microbiome, we will look at both to get a better idea of how they contribute to the aging process.

What Causes Skin Aging?

Skin aging is caused by both intrinsic and extrinsic factors, now also referred to as genetic and epigenetic factors. Causes for intrinsic aging include changes in hormones, immune function, and cellular metabolism as the main factors. Evidence suggests that one major reason our skin ages is the accumulation of what are called senescent (dying) cells. During youth, our immune system seeks out cells that are at the end of their life cycle and eliminates them, making room for new, healthy cells that help keep the infrastructure (proper cell layer ratios and extracellular matrix such as healthy collagen and elastin) of our skin in tip-top shape. However, as we age, something happens. Either there is a change in how our skin's immune cells function, or there is a different expression of genes that help dying cells evade the immune system (or both), so the senescent cells accumulate. Bad news is, when a cell reaches senescence, it becomes inflammatory. That puts aged (and senescent cell-rich) tissue in a chronic state of inflammation without resolution. Dying cells continue to accumulate, more chronic inflammation ensues, and fewer young cells are present to help keep up with the skin infrastructure and additional damage from the extrinsic environmental factors (e.g., UV radiation and free radicals from pollution). All these begin to pile up and take their toll. Add to those factors some physiological changes such as reduced oil/sebum production and reduced hydration levels that result in the physiological changes we see in skin as we age. All these changes in our skin result in a substantial change in the overall skin biome and are accompanied by significant changes in the skin microbiome as well. Skin aging and changes in the skin microbiome are thus highly correlated. But what is the causative agent here? Does aging cause the change in the microbiome, or do changes in the microbiome have anything to do with skin aging? Let's explore.

What do we know about how the skin microbiome affects the aging of skin? One thing we do know is that there are changes to the skin microbiome as we age. These changes seem to be universal. Interestingly, some research has shown that it is so universal that it is possible to predict someone's age, within about four years, by simply looking at the composition of a sample of their skin microbiome. Even more interesting is that the microbiome of the skin is able to do that much more accurately than the microbiome of any other part of the body. What are some of these changes?

Here are a couple of noteworthy changes. There is a striking reduction in the amount of *Cutibacteria* and a notable reduction in the amount of *Staphylococcus* bacteria on the skin of older individuals. As we've discussed, bacteria within those genera—*C. acnes* and *S. epidermidis*—are two of the most important skin commensals for skin health. Another finding that has been reported is that more species of microbes can live on the skin in older individuals, and the changes from site to site on the body become less stark.

So why do these changes happen, and why should we care? It is pretty much agreed thus far that these changes in the skin microbiome are due to physiological and ecological changes to the skin (e.g., less sebum, less hydration), which change the overall skin biome habitats, thus taking away critical food and environmental factors needed to sustain certain microbe communities. Without *C. acnes* and *S. epidermidis* bringing order to the microbiome, more types of microbes can try to move in, and thus there is more diversity. Does this diversity bring about better skin health with regard to aging? While many might argue that more diversity in the microbiome is associated with better skin health, when it comes to aging skin, the answer is no. If it did, we would see skin health go up with age-related microbiome diversity, and we do not. So, it is skin aging that is causative to the changes in the skin microbiome. But do microbiome changes contribute to aging? Let's ask that in a different way. If we attempt to restore the state of the skin microbiome to one of a youthful skin, would that make any difference in the aging process? And here is the rub. If we were a magic 8 ball and you asked us this, we would respond with a resounding, "outlook good!"

As we've discussed, there are many strains of skin commensal species, including *C. acnes* and *S. epidermidis*, and we all have a mixture of many strains of each species. Some are not as helpful, but some are absolute miracle workers in what they do for our skin. In the previous chapter, we saw that protective strains of *C. acnes* produce key skin-healthy substances that tend to stave off issues we see in aging skin. Likewise, protective strains of *S. epidermidis* can have similar effects. Here are just some of the skin benefits we receive by having copious amounts of the protective strains of these microbes on our skin.

We won't rehash all the wonderful things the right strains of microbes can do for the skin when it comes to aging, but it seems that the major microbial constituents of a "younger" skin microbiome, *C. acnes* and *S. epidermidis*, that lessen with age may provide some essential skin-healthy substances that could protect the skin and reduce the signs of aging. The real question is whether a restoration of such a microbiome composition translates to a clinical benefit for aging skin. Can the metabolites from these microbes be anti-aging or de-aging? Can they either prevent further aging or restore youthful attributes to the skin?

While there is much to learn about how a modulation of any given microbiome community affects the host overall, there is quite a bit of evidence that suggests that augmentation of the strains found in more youthful skin would lead to clinical outcomes that mirror more youthful skin. While we know that the body's age comes with changes in the environment that impact our microbiomes, the impact of microbes on aging animal and human cells have been observed to be causative as well, in a positive way. That has been observed when augmenting protective strains of *C. acnes* onto the faces of people who have signs of aging skin such as sagginess, wrinkles, dyspigmentation, unbalanced oil products, and so on. What Dr. Hitchcock and colleagues observed in a study of 130 women was that there were improvements in many of these age-related skin issues in as little as one week after beginning nightly applications. The study subjects who had their skin measured subjectively actually saw continued improvements up to the end of the study—eight weeks of applying *C. acnes defendens*.[5] Given the benefits to skin we are seeing in the clinic with this strategy, curation of the right microbes might be the next anti-aging craze.

Acne

When it comes to the skin microbiome's role in acne, it is no secret that *C. acnes* gets the lion's share of the blame. The species was even named after the disease, so it makes it a convenient scapegoat. Additionally, the use of some antibiotics and other antimicrobials can have some benefit in reducing acne symptoms, leading someone to conclude that *C. acnes* must indeed be behind it all. But one could argue that *C. acnes* should nearly always be present in the development of acne, mainly because the hair follicle (where acne happens) is where *C. acnes* mainly likes to live. Additionally, there is a growing body of evidence that there are other microbial correlations with the occurrence and severity of acne. For instance, the species *S. epidermidis* has been observed to be in higher prevalence in the follicles of those with acne, and the same species has been reported to be more populous in areas where breakouts occur in more severity.[6,7] This does not mean we should rush to any conclusions and pass the blame on to *S. epidermidis* since it is an entire species that (just like *C. acnes*) should not be assumed to be universally equivalent. However, we must admit that there is a correlation that must be explored rather than just defaulting to blaming the *C. acnes* species. To be fair, saying that *C. acnes* is the cause of acne because it is found when swabbing a pimple is like someone blaming you for a burglary in your own home, simply because you were there sleeping at the time it happened. Of course, you were there, it's your home! Sure, you very well may have done it for some reason, but it is worth also exploring the fact that racoons have learned how to navigate their way in and out via the doggy door. You belong in your home, thieving racoons don't. *Cutibacterium acnes* lives in the follicle; *S. epidermidis* normally does not.

While most of those in the know realize that acne is more complicated than simply the presence of certain bacterial strains (i.e., also correlates with hormones, immune cells, and oil production), there is still much misinformation and ambiguity about what is going on. What we must also consider is that those same therapies that are antibacterial can also have both antifungal, anti-inflammatory and keratinolytic properties that can act to modulate the inflammatory state of acne and unblock the follicles as well, both of which are major contributors to acne. This is the case with the go-to topical benzoyl peroxide (BPO). While companies have hung their hat on its ability to kill *C. acnes*, the fact is that there is no evidence that the antimicrobial properties of BPO reduces acne. The FDA has even told companies they can no longer make that claim on their packaging when selling BPO. The reality is that BPO is also strongly antifungal, and has keratolytic and even some anti-inflammatory properties, each of which could equally contribute to how it reduces the severity of acne. It's even now being discovered that the fungal genus *Malassezia*, which is one of the more abundant types of fungus on skin, is more susceptible to BPO than even *C. acnes*.[8] To that end, research is beginning to discover that along with *S. epidermidis* ingress into follicles, the ingress of fungus such as *Malassezia restricta* is also correlated with acne.[9] Regardless, as we have seen here, microbes of both the bacterial and fungal variety do have some correlation with acne. The real question is this: *How* are they correlated? Is it causative or simply correlative?

We know that at puberty we tend to see a larger presence of *C. acnes* on the surface of the skin. We also know that the occurrence of acne tends to increase at puberty. That seems to be a positive correlation (more *C. acnes* correlates to more acne). However, we can then counter that by citing several research publications that state that in the follicular unit (where acne happens), it is actually a relative decrease in the ratio of *C. acnes* to other microbes that is associated with acne. That makes it a negative correlation (less relative *C. acnes* correlates to more acne). It seems that more *C. acnes* correlates to more acne, but at the same time less *C. acnes* correlates to more acne. This is a bit paradoxical, is it not? A caveat here is that it isn't *only C. acnes* that grows more after puberty; it is most of the skin flora that increases in number at that time. More hormones mean more oils which mean more food for microbes, including any skin bacteria and fungus that enjoy those oils as their food source. That is why we tend to have more body odor after puberty, which is due to the sudden increase in Staphylococcus species and apocrine, a certain type of sweat. So, is it the sudden increase in *C. acnes* that causes acne or the overall sudden increase in microflora overall? Conversely, when using antimicrobials to treat acne, is it the targeting and killing of *C. acnes* that alleviates symptoms, or is it the overall reduction of skin bacteria and fungus as a whole that achieves this? While many still believe it is the former, it is likely the latter. That would explain why a *reduction* in relative *C. acnes* would be associated with acne yet a relative reduction in the overall abundance of bacteria (one of which is *C. acnes*) would relieve acne symptoms. That would also lead us to believe that there is some other culprit in the microbiome that is contributing, such as certain strains of *Malasezzia*. This is a bit of potential vindication for *C. acnes*.

We know that certain strains of pathogenic microbes affect both skin cells and immune cells in the skin in ways that make skin more acne-prone such as increasing adhesive molecules in the stratum corneum, increasing porphyrin production, and excess biofilm formation. However, we also know that these pathogenic strains can be found on the skin of those who do *not* have acne. Also, we know that as we age past our teenage years, we are less prone to acne, regardless of whether we continue to have those strains in our microbiome. If it isn't simply a specific strain's presence, what is it? Is it the overgrowth of pathogenic microbes that causes acne as some purport? This is an interesting thought. If a pore gets clogged and provides the *C. acnes* with an oxygen-poor and sebum-rich environment (*C. acnes* heaven), then perhaps that is the case.

Let's explore that. What are some of the reasons *C. acnes* might overgrow? And if it does overgrow, will that truly lead to acne?

Excess oils/sebum: As we already said, the phenomenon of a significant increase in oil/sebum secretion at puberty is somewhat universal although more significant for some than others. That, of course, will lead to a significant increase in the number of overall bacteria growing in those areas that are more sebaceous or oily since oil/sebum is the "nectar of the gods" for some skin microbes such as *C. acnes*. With any sudden change to the flora in the skin biome, it makes sense that the innate immune system would take note and react accordingly to (1) the increased number of what is "moving in" to the area and (2) to make sure everything is under control. We see this with newborns who experience baby acne (erythema toxicum neonatorum), which is thought to be an activation of the immune system in the skin due to the sudden appearance of foreign microbes—well, at least more microbes—since there are definitely more types and more of all types of microbes outside the womb. Once the immune system recognizes that these microbes are friendly, the condition subsides.

Acne at puberty isn't as simple to explain, and it can follow someone around for quite a while. Why is that? It isn't just an increase in oil production that happens spontaneously during puberty; it is the introduction of androgens—good ol' hormones—that cause all sorts of changes to the body, not just increases in oil secretion. They are also responsible for changing how our immune system functions. Research has found that increases in testosterone and estrogen can help reduce immune predisposition to inflammation. On the other hand, estrogen can also be associated with induction of autoimmune issues. How are both possible? Could it be that the fluctuation in hormones throughout the day, week, or month can lead to changes to the immune cells' proclivity to cause issues against our own skin and skin microbiome? Perhaps. Female hormones could be one of the reasons females tend to have acne more often and longer into their adult lives.

We know that it can't just be an overproduction of oils that lead to acne via overgrowth of *C. acnes*, because there are many people that struggle with very oily skin and do not have acne. Actually, it might even be said that oily skin ages better. Let's think about one of the hallmarks of acne, the blackhead. We normally have collections of substances in our follicles, some of which help to keep the follicle clear of microbes that can cause issues. However, blackheads are created when there is an accumulation of sebum in the follicle that produces a filament that is unusually large and visible. To top it off, the oxidation of the large sebaceous filament then turns it dark in color, making it even more obvious (and thus the name *black* head). So, if acne is caused by *C. acnes* overgrowth, then how is it that blackheads exist? If sebum is the *C. acnes* preferred meal, then overgrowth of *C. acnes* should colonize and digest any filament long before it turns any color! Additionally, if the blackhead is plugging the pore, why does this not become inflamed? Is this another paradox?

Dr. Hitchcock: *The paradox of the existence of blackheads in acneic skin did give me some pause in the past. Given that C. acnes is supposed to be unusually proliferative and prefers the skin sebum/oils as a food source, we would think that a proliferation of C. acnes would actually reduce the amount, or at least the size, of sebaceous plugs in the skin. To explore this in my lab, we ran a small pilot clinical study where we applied three trillion C. acnes bacteria every night to the faces of a number of individuals, myself included, with different skin types. Interestingly, no one had any increases in acneic symptoms such as redness, pimples or comedones (blackheads or whiteheads). In fact, in the two individuals who presented with blackheads, there was a significant reduction in the size and appearance of the blackheads following three weeks of nightly applications. This is when I became convinced that to blame acne on the species of C. acnes was reductive and the true driving force behind the skin issue needed to be revisited.*

The reality is that a simple overgrowth of *C. acnes* due to increased oil production being the cause of acne is correlative, but it is ambiguous as to whether or at least *how* it is causative. While we are on this subject, we also wanted to learn if there is a threshold of overgrowth of *C. acnes* that is supposed to cause acne. Dr. Hitchcock conducted another study where 108 subjects applied 100 billion *C. acnes defendens* each night for eight weeks. The study found that after applying literally *billions* of *C. acnes* bacteria to the face every night, not one acne lesion was reported. How can we simply point to *C. acnes* overgrowth as a cause of acne? It just cannot be that simple.

In Dr. Hitchcock's study, only one strain of *C. acnes* was used—a protective strain known not to be highly associated with acne. Other researchers have reported that other strains considered pathogenic can cause the production of inflammatory cytokines in the skin and contribute potentially to the inflammatory nature of acne. However, many (if not most) of those pathogenic *C. acnes* can also be found on the skin of those who do not have acne. What we do know is that some strains of *C. acnes* are more associated with acne than others. However, an association (correlation) does not imply causation. We still need to show how a *C. acnes* strain thought to be pathogenic (more associated with acne) might actually cause acne. After all, we all have large amounts of *C. acnes* in our skin, and there are many strains (not just one or two) on all of us. So it is not simply the strain of *C. acnes* that is important but also the predisposition to acne of the person whose skin the strains are on. The real question is why some strains are more associated with *C. acnes*. That leads us to our next potential causative link to acne: clogging of pores.

Clogged pores: How exactly does a pore get clogged? Is it like your sink? Can you place topicals on the skin that literally clog your pores, or is it something that instigates other mechanisms that lead to clogged pores? In reference to pimple formation, the term *pore clogging* is a bit of a misnomer. While excess sebum and *C. acnes* biofilm can accumulate in the hair follicles/pores, leading to blackheads (or open comedones), that isn't truly a blockage. Most of the time, they are usually easily extracted. However, a pimple appears not when a pore is clogged but when the outermost layer of skin, the stratum corneum, overgrows (called hyper-keratinization), thus sealing in the contents of the pore. Once the pore is sealed, the sebum accumulates and the oxygen content lowers, which makes a perfect environment for the resident *C. acnes* to thrive. While some strains of *C. acnes* can produce irritating molecules that may accumulate and further inflame the pimple, we are learning that this may not be what starts the process.

In a 1981 article by Robert M. Lavker, Ph.D., James J. Leyden, M.D., and Kenneth J. McGinley, it was shown that in almost pubescent children, abnormal keratinization (pore clogging) is already beginning to happen without the prompt from sebum production and *C. acnes* overgrowth.[10] However, this is contradicted in a more recent publication that claims that *C. acnes* causes hyperkeratinization by causing skin cells to secrete an excess of skin barrier molecules.[11] However, the latter study only used one strain of *C. acnes* (likely disease associated) and did not use live strains, leading us to wonder if what they observed was a combination of the wrong strain and artifacts caused by experimental design.

Regardless of whether *C. acnes* plays a role in the sealing of pores and pimple formation, we know it is not a direct cause since there is much evidence that people can have even the disease-associated strains on or in their skin and not have acne.[12] It is the inflammation and immune cell imbalance that effectively causes the sealing of the pore, or the clogging. This can also be driven by fungal species as we alluded to earlier.

How to Calm a Perfect Storm: We hope that by now it is evident that it is not simply the presence of any particular species or strains of microbes on the skin that is *the* cause of acne. However, we can definitely say that they contribute to the disease state. You may wonder why this is an important distinction. The importance lies in the means by which we try to treat a disease state such as acne. If we continue to overemphasize the use of antimicrobials to treat acne, we are left forever running in circles, hoping to bide time and soften the effects until someone ages out of the disease. However, Dr. Day sees patients daily who are living with acne as adults, trying every antimicrobial there is, with little to no respite. They are often hesitant to stop the antibiotics for fear of a flare of their acne and it often takes much convincing to help her patients understand that long-term use of antibiotics is unhealthy and is not the answer. Fortunately, there are alternatives. In her practice, Dr. Day has now reduced oral antibiotic use by close to 100%, with even better and long-lasting clearance of acne in her patients by focusing more on restoring a healthy skin biome and using a more biome friendly and supportive approach.

If we look at disease states such as acne as a sort of perfect storm where we need to treat several facets of the disease in order to truly cure it, we are much more likely to find success. We will discuss the Biomecare strategy for treating acne in Chapters 7 and 8.

ATOPIC DERMATITIS/ECZEMA

Atopic dermatitis (AD), also known as eczema, is a common inflammatory skin disease that can affect almost any population, although it has been documented to affect some populations more than others. One study observed an overall disease prevalence for children to be 10.7% of the population in the United States. The study also found that those who lived in urban areas had a significantly higher prevalence of AD, as did those whose guardians had more than a post-secondary education.[13] Another study from the National Health and Nutrition Examination Survey stated that African-American children had the highest rate of AD prevalence (19.3%), followed by Caucasian children (16.1%) and Asian children (7.8%). In a separate study, it was found that adults have a slightly lower incidence rate of AD (7.2%) in the United States.[14] Interestingly, while there were some similarities in the adult demographics that tend to have a higher prevalence of AD (such as a post-secondary education), there were some disparities such as lower association with African-American adults. Other distinguishing factors that were less associated with AD were higher household income (over

$75K/year), families with children (especially more than one), and a birthplace outside the United States. One noteworthy observation in adults was that a body mass index (BMI) of 35 or more was also associated with a higher prevalence of AD. Also, there is often an association between AD and food allergies and asthma.[15,16] That last predisposition is thought to be due to an impaired skin barrier function that allows potential allergens to penetrate the skin and promote systemic allergen sensitization.

When we look at many of these factors that affect our potential to have AD, it is not intuitive why some of them may contribute. Why would African-American children have a higher prevalence and their parents a lower prevalence? Why would those with a higher education have a higher prevalence but those with a higher income have a lower prevalence? To begin to answer this, we need to look at the known contributors to the disease, as well as the correlations to the skin microbiome.

Like acne, the pathogenesis of AD is not straightforward and can include a mixture of both genetic, environmental and microbiome constituents. The hallmarks of the disease state are an altered skin barrier, higher skin pH, immune dysregulation, and a higher prevalence of *S. aureus*.[17] Despite these hallmarks, there are subgroups or types of AD that all have different clinical characteristics.[18] However, whichever form AD takes, it all starts with a predisposition of the innate and adaptive immune cells to be in an inflammatory state and the skin barrier to be disrupted. Ironically, these two things can influence one another and lead to more severe disease. The last ingredient of the disease state is the composition of the microbiome; namely, an increased burden of certain strains of *Staphylococcus aureus* on the affected skin, especially in more severely affected skin.

Both genetic issues (immune dysfunction and impaired skin barrier) and the dysbiosis of the skin microbiome are positively correlated with AD. But which, is the cause? Again, as was the case of acne and *C. acnes*, we have a bit of a chicken and egg situation. We know that certain genetic predispositions lend to disruption of the skin barrier and a pro-inflammatory inclination such as the gene FLG that codes for the filaggrin protein essential for skin barrier health.[19] Such disruptions in the skin barrier can make it easier for the entry of pathogens into the skin, which can then activate the immune system and thus lead to further inflammation.

What about the microbial contributions to AD? It has been observed that in those with AD, the amount of total bacteria on the skin tends to increase. Interestingly, so do some of the fungal strains such as *Candida albicans*, but very little is known about how this contributes to the disease.[20] However, although the microbes go up, a reported trend is for those with AD to have dysbiosis in the form of *less* microbial diversity on the skin overall (and interestingly in the gut as well). However, it has been observed that when the total microbial burden goes up on the skin, while *S. aureus* amounts go up, the commensals such as *C. acnes* stay the same.[21] It is notable that in the most severe AD lesions, the *Corynebacterium* and *Cutibacterium* species have been seen to be significantly fewer in numbers compared to those without AD.[22] And it isn't simply the increase in *S. aureus* that is the issue. As with *C. acnes*, there are numerous strains of *S. aureus*, and we are still learning what that means for the skin microbiome. In this case with AD, researchers have seen that certain strains of *S. aureus* seem to be more pathogenic than others. This means that the *S. aureus* that is taken from people who have AD can induce inflammation on skin when transplanted more so than *S. aureus* taken from the skin of people without AD.[23,24]

And it is not only the strain differences in *S. aureus* that might contribute to AD. It is also the strain differences in commensals such as *S. epidermidis* and *S. hominis* that can fail to protect the skin. While *S. aureus* overgrowth tends to be a hallmark of AD lesions, the commensals tend to dominate the skin that does not contain lesions on AD sufferers.[25] What has been observed is that commensal strains from those without AD are more often able to kill *S. aureus* compared to commensals taken from those with AD.[26] So just like with acne, the strains involved with AD are strain-specific and may not be a direct cause for the disease state alone but act in tandem with the human predisposition to the disease state.

Thus, it seems to be a vicious cycle where skin barrier deficiencies lead to more colonization with more pathogenic *S. aureus* strains, which through secretion of enterotoxins and other inflammatory factors can perpetuate an inflammatory skin state that leads to immune cell recruitment, further barrier impairment, and microbiome dysbiosis . . . and thus it repeats. Since AD sufferers tend to have less diversity of the microbiome of the gut as well, it is likely that such an inflammatory cycle may also be perpetuating in the gut and contributing to this state.

Using this knowledge, we will discuss in Chapter 7 the Biomecare strategy to fight atopic dermatitis.

Skin Cancer

While scientists don't yet have a firm understanding of the connection of the skin microbiome to skin cancers such as squamous cell carcinoma (SCC) and melanoma or precancers such as actinic keratosis (AK), there have been some recognizable correlations. For instance, when looking at the skin of men who are predisposed to AK and SCC, it was found that the *Cutibacterium* and *Malassezia* species were relatively more prevalent in nonlesional photodamaged skin than on the actual cancerous or precancerous lesions themselves. On the flip side, the *Staphylococcus* species was most commonly associated with the lesions—in particular, *Staphylococcus aureus*.[27] Given the associations we have discussed with skin health and skin issues such as atopic dermatitis, the association of these strains with both health and cancer is not really a surprise. However, we must then ask whether or not strains such as *S. aureus* and their correlation with skin cancers is a causative one. And it isn't just bacteria; there are associations of certain viruses such as human papillomaviruses that play an important role in skin cancer development.

Lessons from the GI Microbiome and Cancer: Whether microbes play a causative role in the development of skin cancers is a tricky question. We know there are strong associations of certain microbes with skin cancers, especially in the gut microbiome. An example of this is the microbe *Heliobacter pylori*, a species of microbe that is very much associated with cancers in the GI tract. This is thought to be due to the chronic inflammation that *H. pylori* produces in the gut, leading to GI issues such as ulcers. An interesting note about *H. pylori* is that some reports show that the species can be protective against some forms of cancer (esophageal and pancreatic). That may come across as contradictory, but if you recall from our discussion on *C. acnes*, we are finding that a single species can have quite a community of strains that can have both pathogenic and protective members. Additionally, the environment the strains grow in can affect how they act and what they secrete, so even the same strain can interact differently with the human host, depending on where it is located, what other microbes are around it, and what nutrients are available, among other factors.

Microbe-Associated Inflammation May Have a Role: There are many similarities in how the skin microbiome and the gut microbiome interact with the human host. Both the skin and the gut are considered the largest immune organs (or groups of organs), although it is debated which one is actually the largest. Regardless, both contain epithelial cells that come into direct contact with trillions of microbes at any given moment and thus require critical regulation in order to keep the biome in order. As we have already discussed, when the biome of any organ becomes dysbiotic, it can lead to all sorts of inflammatory issues. While a small amount of inflammation is not typically worrisome, it has been observed that chronic tissue injury and unregulated inflammation is highly associated with the formation of many types of cancers, both in the gut and the skin.[28,29] An example of this is burn scars, 2% of which form skin cancers.[30]

Since the skin microbiome has a huge role in regulating skin inflammation and modulating the immune system, we must realize that the connection between the microbes of the skin and cancers of the skin are not insignificant. Regardless of the actual connection, chronic inflammatory skin issues such as acne and psoriasis have a high association with cancer formation,[31] and the links of certain species (e.g., *S. aureus* and SCC) of microbes to cancer are undeniable.

The microbes in the gut and cancer of the gut are typically connected by specific inflammatory pathways. These same pathways are involved with inflammatory skin issues such as acne, atopic dermatitis, and psoriasis, so it stands to reason that when these become unbalanced, they can lead to cancer formation[32,33,34] just like in the GI tract. Evidence has been found that these pathways are associated since skin cancers such as melanoma and basal cell carcinoma can be treated successfully by blocking these inflammatory pathways.[35] However, we do need these pathways to be active since they cause the immune system to scan the skin and destroy any pathogens or cancerous cells that may be forming. Just like with other inflammatory skin issues, we do not need a complete mitigation of inflammation, but simply need to get to a more normal balance. We can think of it as a light switch versus a dimmer switch—rather than on-off, we simply want to decrease the light. Our commensal and symbiotic microbes on the skin can do that naturally, by interacting with specific cells in the skin immune community (e.g., T-regulatory cells) that turn on the surveillance system of the skin and protect against cancers.

In Chapter 7, we will discuss the Biomecare strategy to reduce the potential for skin cancers, including how microbes can best be used to potentially fight skin cancers.

OUR HABITS AND HOW THEY AFFECT BIOME BALANCE

In this chapter, we have covered a few skin issues that have correlations with the skin microbiome, including aging, acne, atopic dermatitis, and cancer, but this list is by no means exhaustive. However, there is commonality among them. Microbes may be that connection. This means that the role of the skin microbiome should be a major focus for anyone who is interested in the health and beauty of the skin. We need to make sure we take care of the skin's environment since that is a major driver for the microbes that take up residence on our skin. To that end, it is important to take special care when considering what we put on our skin when it comes to hygiene, skin care, and even medicine. Substances such as benzoyl peroxide (BPO) can be great tools to help get acne under control; however, the free radicals it produces in the skin make the way it is used critical. That is why BPO washes make the most sense since reductions of inflammation and clogged pores with any free radicals produced are kept mostly at the superficial layer (stratum corneum) and are less likely to affect the long-term health of the skin. Leaving on BPO, on the other hand, is riskier. You can run the risk of skin cell toxicity. Likewise, antibiotics play a huge role in medicine but are often abused and can lead not only to dysbiosis of the skin and gut microbiome but also to the emergence of resistant strains.

Finally, keep in mind that we are just starting to understand the importance of the skin microbiome and how the topicals we use affect them and thus our own skin biology. This is an evolving science, and as we learn more, we will be able to improve treatments and outcome, which is how science and medicine work together. It is now time to realize that it is the entire biome we must care for, not just the skin. If we keep that in mind, our choices will eventually lead us in the right direction. Remember, the point of this book is to allow us to know better so we can do better.

CHAPTER 5

A PROBIOTIC BY ANY OTHER NAME

The whole is greater than the sum of its parts.
—Aristotle

One way the Holobiont Philosophy is different from traditional skin care is in the comprehensive way it considers and includes the skin biome in any diagnosis or treatment. Skin biome care that follows this philosophy doesn't look at caring for the skin as independent from caring for its microbiome; both aspects are equally as important since they are inextricably linked. When it comes to looking at the ingredients we want to include in our daily topical regimens, it is best to look at all ingredients through the scope of this philosophy. Ask yourself this: "Will this benefit *both* my skin and its symbiotic microbes?" That is important since there is a myriad of ingredients available that tout benefits, usually found by observing how skin cells react to them in a Petri dish or other artificial, isolated condition. When we look at a laundry list of ingredients for any topical, we need to ask if they are tested to see if they impart a benefit to the skin biome, or at least not harm it. Knowing the answers to these questions is important when it comes to the inclusion and marketing of the microbiome-related terms *prebiotic*, *probiotic*, and *postbiotic*. Let's see why the simple inclusion of these terms on a list of marketing claims may not mean what you think it does or do what you hope it will.

Most consumers have little idea what *probiotics* are, why they need them, or what they should look for to find a legitimate probiotic that works. It can be very confusing; even in gut health where consumers are a bit more savvy, there is a myriad of vague labels and claims purporting more strains, better strains but a dearth of consumer facing information what this all means or whether it is even really important. Then there are the related terms *prebiotics* and *postbiotics* that are beginning to become more common on product labels, but their relevance is still under investigation, even to scientists. Consumers may want to improve their health through evidence-based science rather than marketing gimmicks, but most time they have no idea where to begin in choosing the best products with true efficacy. This is even truer for the recent emergence of skin topical products that use the monikers of probiotic, prebiotic and postbiotic while their ingredients only loosely reflect the actual definitions of those terms.

In this chapter, we will explain everything you need to know about probiotics, prebiotics, and postbiotics, as well as the science behind using microbes and microbe-derived products for the health and balance of your skin. We will discuss some dubious ways microbe-containing or microbe-derived products are already being marketed in the skin care arena and how, while the awareness of the microbiome is a good thing, we need to be careful not to fall prey to gimmicks that often become prevalent when it comes to any new, hot topic such as the skin microbiome where profit is sometimes placed above science.

PROBIOTICS: CURATED PROTECTIVE MICROBES

There is an emerging trend for everyday skin care products to claim some form of microbiome-friendly or microbiome-gentle designation which refers to how those products do or do not interfere with the innate balance of the skin microbiome. Because there are no current regulatory standards for measuring if a product is microbiome-gentle, friendly, or safe, companies are left to define these terms for themselves. As the number of products in this category begins to increase, regulation may follow, but until then, we will guide you to the truly beneficial products that enhance and support your skin's natural biome so you can help your skin stay healthy and age beautifully.

Many products that call themselves microbiome-friendly, safe, or gentle do not actively make the skin microbiome composition worse, but they also do not necessarily make it better. These are products that are formulated pretty much as any typical topical would be, albeit, using ingredients that have been tested not to be harmful with the skin microbes. However, it isn't just how "friendly" a topical or its ingredients are that is matters, the two most important points to consider are:

- How the topical affects the environment of the skin biome

- This will in turn affect which microbes thrive, how fast they grow, and what substances (helpful or harmful) they secrete

Another strategy is to create products whose formulas contain ingredients can interact directly with or to use elements of the microbiome itself to make the skin biome healthier, and more balanced. Products that adopt this strategy typically act on the skin biome through microbes, microbe-derived ingredients and microbe-related ingredients. One of those being touted as probiotics. But what we still need to discuss is what exactly constitutes a probiotic when it comes to topical skin biome care.

The definition of the word *probiotic* has evolved over time and is still somewhat ambiguous within the discipline. The term commonly refers to bacteria that are beneficial to our health. The World Health Organization defines probiotics as "live microorganisms that, when administered in adequate amounts, confer a health benefit on the host." However, in common vernacular, the word typically refers to the use of a microbe (typically a bacterium) for therapeutic purposes. But there are considerations as to what makes a microbe therapeutic. Much of that is dependent on the environment in which any given microbe is placed. Placing a microbe in one specific area might be neutral or beneficial, while placing it in another area can be harmful and even lead to infection.

With regard to the skin, the definition of *probiotic* becomes even more nuanced. You might assume that products labeled probiotic for gut health could be adapted for skin health as well, but it doesn't work that way because the strains that are beneficial for the skin are not the same as those that are good for the gut. Not surprisingly, the gut and the skin microbiomes are made up of significantly different organisms, require different environments, and utilize different food sources. Which organisms, then, are considered a true skin probiotic?

When we consider the gut microbiome, we can go to the local grocery store and find any number of products that claim some sort of probiotic benefit. Some are refrigerated, and some are not. Some contain prebiotics, and some do not. They typically have a long list of strains that mainly consist of gut- or dairy-related *Lactobacillus* and *Bifidobacterium* strains such as *Lactobacillus acidophilus, Lactobacillus casei, Lactobacillus reuteri,* and *Bifidobacterium lactis.* This list is far from exhaustive. Some of the strains commonly found in these products have been studied longer and have more scientific and even clinical support when it comes to potential health benefits for the digestive system. Yet it has been found that the benefits of probiotic organisms can't always be attributed to a whole microbial species but often are specific to a subspecies or even a specific strain within that subspecies. Some of the strains used in products can be somewhat gimmicky since they are not known to confer much, if any, health benefits. They are simply thrown in to give the optics of more diversity (a common mantra in the microbiome ethos) though not always relevant, as we discussed in Chapter 3.

Companies simply want to have a longer list of strains in their ingredients to appeal to our psychological assumption that more equals better. You commonly see these kinds of tactic: "*If 38 billion live cultures is good, then 58 billion must be better!" "Are 10 strains good? Then 18 strains must be better!*" While it is generally agreed upon that some gut health probiotic strains can be quite helpful for certain indications, just because a product carries the moniker "probiotic" doesn't necessarily make it beneficial to your health, given the current lack of standards and regulations in the supplement industry. There are considerations other than what strain it contains, such as whether or not it is actually living and how it's been stored, which can have a huge impact on whether the probiotics are capable of imparting some of their benefits or any at all. Some companies that are legit will provide proof of these things, which helps give confidence to the consumer.

When it comes to skin health, companies are scrambling to jump on the biome bandwagon. Since probiotics for gut health have been around so long and the infrastructure to produce gut-related bacteria strains is established and commoditized, many skin care ingredient manufacturers have adopted them in their portfolios and are pushing them to skin care companies, purporting that it will allow them to make probiotic claims for their skin care products. But there are some issues with that strategy that we need to discuss.

When you look at the majority of skin-related products on the market that claim some sort of probiotic ingredient, you find that they typically fall into a few of the following categories:

1. Live gut or dairy-related strains

2. Dead gut or dairy-related strains, or pieces of such

3. Lysates (the guts of a bacteria, if you will)

4. Ferments of gut- or dairy-related strains (actually postbiotics, which we will discuss later in this chapter)

The issue lies not in the fact that the ingredients are used in topical products but that they are being referred to as probiotic, which they are not. Simply consisting of a microbe or parts of a microbe does not mean something is probiotic. If that were the case, then using the pathogenic MRSA or flesh-eating bacteria on the face could be considered probiotic (note: please don't do that). Why, then, would or should gut- or dairy-related microbes or their parts be considered a probiotic when used in skin care? What is the rationale for why a gut-related microbe would be useful to improve the health or beauty of skin?

To answer this, let's consider a few ideas. Firstly, microbes that reside in the microbiomes of various areas of the body must find that area of the body hospitable in order to engraft there and exert any type of long-term influence or benefit. Gut-related bacteria such as the *Lactobacillus* species are plentiful in the gut, mouth, and vagina but are not found on the skin in any appreciable amount. The skin of the face is a much different ecosystem than that of the gut, mouth or vagina; they all have different temperatures, different food sources for microbes, different pH, and so on. If we think of the skin as an ecosystem, we can make the analogy that you wouldn't try planting a banana tree in Antarctica because they are great for feeding monkeys in tropical areas. Monkeys don't live in Antarctica, and even if they did, a banana tree wouldn't live long enough to feed them. So why would it make sense to use gut microbes that are not able to live and function properly on the skin?

Some experimental models have shown that some gut-related strains such as *Lactobacillus reuteri* may secrete substances that have benefits to skin, purporting anti-inflammatory and even antimicrobial properties. However, there is little to no evidence that these benefits are possible outside of a Petri dish. If the microbe placed on the skin cannot live there in any appreciable amount for any appreciable time, then it cannot in any appreciable way produce the substances that are being claimed as beneficial. A microbe outside its niche is basically a banana tree in Antarctica. It may be able to survive for a short time, but then it is gone along with any potential benefits.

While live gut bacteria for the skin may not make the most sense, pieces of these strains (called lysates) could have some benefit when used as skin care ingredients. The question becomes whether or not these components will produce effects that are good for the skin. For example, certain parts of some bacterial strains can cause inflammatory (negative) reactions in human cells such as the inflammatory effects induced in human cells by lipopolysaccharides found in bacterial cell walls. Other specific lysates have been shown in laboratories to be effective in reducing inflammation, limiting UV damage, and repairing barriers. That may mimic results we're already getting from existing skin care products, but the growing demand for probiotics has led for a push to include such lysates in order to claim a topical is a "microbiome" technology. A lysate from a non-skin microbe may provide some benefits as an ingredient (as long as the parts that are inflammatory have been removed), but this does not make it a "microbiome" product, probiotic or postbiotic. It is simply an ingredient.

The bastardization of the terms probiotic, prebiotic and postbiotic have led to the need for stricter requirements for scientific evidence of probiotic benefit claims. In a 2015 publication titled "Selective Manipulation of the Gut Microbiota Improves Immune Status in Vertebrates," the authors describe what most researchers in the field consider the characteristics that a microbe should have in order to be considered a true probiotic. The authors state that probiotics must do the following:

1. Have the capacity to survive in the relevant area of the body they are to be used in

2. Display a high resistance to any environmental stressors specific to that location

3. Lack any transferable antibiotic-resistant gene

4. Be able to confer clear benefits to the host through the modulation of the resident microbiome

5. Be non-pathogenic and non-toxic, and provide protection against disease-causing microorganisms by means of multiple inherent mechanisms.

At the time of writing this book very few brands that boast the probiotic claim actually meet these requirements; however, a select few are emerging. One of which was founded by Dr. Hitchcock and developed over 9 years in his own labs. This brand, called BIOJUVE, follows the holobiont philosophy, using a skin-related strain that adheres to the above definition of a legitimate skin probiotic. And that is no small feat. As you can imagine, finding skin-relevant strains that meet the requirements to be truly considered skin probiotics is one thing; it is quite another to invest in an infrastructure to produce those strains and develop formulations that allow them to remain stable for an acceptable amount of time to be used by the general population.

These are indeed hurdles that need to be overcome in order to bring novel and effective true skin probiotic technologies to the market. And while most companies have opted to take the easy (and somewhat pseudoscientific) route, there are at least a couple organizations that have invested in an infrastructure to bring true skin biome science to consumers.

PREBIOTICS: NOT JUST THE FOOD OF THE MICROBES BUT THE *RIGHT* FOOD

Just as probiotics have gained popularity in gut health and now increasingly in skin health, the term *prebiotic* is also popping up at mainstream health food stores, grocery stores, and more. But how are prebiotics different from probiotics, and are the benefits different?

Prebiotics are quite simply substances that foster the health and activity of your beneficial microflora. In essence, they are the opposite of an antibiotic. For the gut, prebiotics are mostly comprised of fiber compounds that cannot be digested by humans and are touted for their positive benefits to your gut microbiome and thus gut health. Most people think about it simply as the food of the probiotic microbes. However, they are much more than that. While having the right food source is critical for the health of a microbe, having the right environment is just as important. Equally important is that prebiotics should provide both a food source and an environment that is conducive to the growth and function of only beneficial, or commensal, microbes while discouraging growth of pathogenic microbes. That is true in the gut *and* the skin. For instance, quite a few bacteria on the skin can eat carbohydrates such as glucose or sugar, but unfortunately so can the pathogenic microbes such as MRSA. However, MRSA requires a much higher pH environment to thrive than the beneficial flora of the skin does. A food source such as glucose (sugar) might cause growth of all bacteria on the skin, even MRSA, especially if the pH of the skin is elevated by over washing. The combination of an agnostic food source and high pH would essentially be the opposite of a prebiotic; it would be a *prepathotic* (or feeding the pathogen, if you allow us to coin a term) that would boost the growth of pathogenic microbes by providing an ideal environment for their growth. A true prebiotic would be an ingredient that either preferentially feeds a good microbe, provides an environment biased toward the good microbe, or both. To carry our example forward, a true skin prebiotic would lower pH appropriately, like fatty acids that are produced by *C. acnes* metabolism and serve to lower pH (among other things), so it will not only foster growth of beneficial microbes, including true skin probiotics, but will also keep pathogens such as MRSA at bay.

As we discussed earlier, a true skin probiotic would be a microbe that can survive and thrive on the skin and impart a skin health benefit. To do that, a true skin probiotic must find the environment and food sources available on the skin (e.g., low pH, sebum, fatty acids, sweat) acceptable. *So, we could extrapolate that the qualities that already exist on healthy skin might make the best prebiotic.*

Prebiotics your skin naturally makes:

- Skin oils, sebum

- Sweat

- Keratin (the proteins that make up your skin cells)

In other words, your skin already makes some of the best prebiotic ingredients for your skin microflora. That is one reason modern-day grooming habits can at times err on the side of *too* clean. Getting that squeaky clean feeling, peeling off pore strips, using pore vacuums, and constant aggressive exfoliation are included in the skin care habits that really mess with the skin's microenvironment that a microbiome needs in order to help keep the skin biome healthy and balanced.

So, take it easy on the skin when you groom. Use gentle soap on those key parts that might need a bit more cleansing (we all know which bits those are), but simply use water on the rest such as your extremities (as long as they aren't soiled). You will find that it is quite adequate for most days and will help keep your skin barrier in better shape and reduce the need for topical moisturizers on those areas in order to maintain hydration. Keep the use of products and procedures that disrupt the normal architecture of the skin (aggressive exfoliators, pore strips) to a minimum, and replace them with microbiome-friendly products that have ingredients such as salicylic acid and retinyl propionate that gently achieve the same if not better results when used strategically. You can still pamper your skin without significantly disrupting your skin biome. Trust us, your skin will thank you.

POSTBIOTICS: MORE THAN JUST A PROBIOTIC'S POO

If you turn over a container of skin care and see the word *ferment* on the ingredient list, you've likely found a product with *post*biotics. That might be confusing because many examples of skin care that claim they contain probiotics actually contain postbiotics in the form of either bacterial ferment (the "soup" that bacteria has grown in and released metabolites into) or a bacterial lysate (the contents in a bacterial cell). Think of cracking open an egg. The lysate is like everything inside, and sometimes you can throw in the shell, depending on who you ask. Postbiotics are typically defined as the metabolites of microbes that are beneficial to the health of the host. Many mistakenly reduce the term to simply mean the waste products of microbes—or to put in crass terms, "bacteria's poo." A postbiotic is much more than that. It's true that during certain strains' metabolic processes, some substances can be created that are undesirable. An example is the metabolism of apocrine sweat (the sweat produced under the arms, especially when nervous) by certain *Staph* species that can result in byproducts we identify as body malodor. Would we call such substances postbiotics? Probably not unless we can determine that they create some sort of benefit to the host. At the time of writing this, we don't believe we are aware of evidence that the after-gym smell has been proven to be beneficial to anyone, especially your loved ones.

Not only waste products of probiotics, postbiotics can be quite a complex mixture of substances, from small molecules to enzymes that a microbe might secrete *either* as a byproduct of metabolism *or* as a means for important biological functions to establish their niche in the microbiome and often to protect itself. Keep in mind too that just because a substance from a microbe is a byproduct of metabolism doesn't mean it isn't beneficial. An example of this is the postbiotics created by our good friend *C. acnes defendens*, which you now know as one of the main beneficial subspecies of *C. acnes*. These little guys have been shown to secrete a complex mixture of metabolites, including substances that are anti-inflammatory in nature such as fatty acids that modulate skin pH and powerful antioxidants that allow this facultative anaerobe oxygen-phobic microbe to venture out to the skin's surface and still thrive. Not only has all this been observed in Dr. Hitchcock's research but also in the labs of several other well-respected scientists, including Huiying Li of UCLA and Richard Gallo of UCSD. The postbiotic that *C. acnes defendens* produces protects them *and* your skin at the same time. As a result, the more *C. acnes defendens* there are on the skin, the more the skin's oils are filled with skin-healthy substances.

However, the metabolites of microbes are extremely strain specific. They are also specific to the environment and food source the microbe receives. A microbe that is grown in a commercial fermenter and is only given glucose as a carbon source may produce a very different postbiotic profile than a microbe that grows in the soil or on the skin. Scientists are exploring how to produce the fermented products with the best constituents so they can put them in products and provide the greatest benefit for the skin. There is a so-called secret formula to proper fermentation that leads to truly beneficial postbiotics. Unfortunately, it means that when you read your skin care ingredients you **cannot assume that all ferments from the same strains of microbes are equal.** That is when you really need to do your homework and make sure the skin care company has done its homework. In essence, you should look for clinical research that proves that the ferment that particular company is using comes from a process that has been proven to provide benefit. Otherwise, all you can do is trust.

As we discussed previously, while attempting to place a *Lactobacillus* strain on your face may not make the most sense because it would have a hard time engrafting, the ferment of certain Lactobacillus species has been studied and suggested to contain skin-healthy substances that can help with skin health. But we need to be careful about assuming that all lysates and ferments are good for the skin. As mentioned, lysates can also contain pieces of microbial cell walls such as lipopolysaccharides (LPS). They can be inflammatory and potentially reduce or even negate any benefit from other components of the lysate. Additionally, ferment products of certain microbes can be quite toxic (do cholera and botulism ring a bell?). We don't think most companies would dare use anything so ridiculous in their products but doesn't mean they won't though, so be sure to read those labels! And of course, it's always a good idea to run new products past your dermatologist.

The good news is that if a microbe is a true probiotic, it likely produces a postbiotic of some form (depending on what the manufacturer fed the microbe or microbes). When you see a ferment or lysate in your skin care, look at the strain and see whether it is a strain that would be considered a probiotic. Then determine if it is a company you trust that curates their ingredients to make sure they have science behind them and are not just gimmicks. That will help you determine if the postbiotic product is something you want to spend your hard-earned dollars on and, even more importantly, if you even want to put it on your skin.

THE WHOLE IS GREATER

In this chapter, we have discussed exactly what prebiotics, probiotics, and postbiotics are—or at least how they are defined since the terms have become somewhat bastardized in recent years. However, we must now ask ourselves this: What is the point of using these three types of ingredients when it comes to the health of our skin biome? Is there some species of microbe in the world that our skin doesn't already harbor that can impart such significant effects that it is worth the effort to try to feign or force engraftment in order to harvest their benefits? Or does our own skin already contain the secrets of the truest and best forms of prebiotics, probiotics, and postbiotics? That is not to say that perhaps we might not need a bit of help to curate the right *strains* of microbes in our skin biome or maximize the benefits of our skin biome. However, we leave you with the thought that it is not simply a random or even a select yet agnostic mishmash of prebiotics, probiotics, and postbiotics that confer the best health for the skin biome. These are just the parts. It is the *whole* that is essential. This is reflected in the cyclical nature of an optimal skin environment (prebiotic) that fosters the right microbes (probiotic) that produce all the skin-healthy substances (postbiotics) that make for an optimal skin biome environment—and repeat. This is the epitome of the Holobiont Philosophy.

CHAPTER 6

CONSUMER CLICKBAIT: MARKETING THE MICROBIOME

All marketers are storytellers. Only the losers are liars.
—Seth Godin

Even if we do not consider ourselves "salespeople" as a profession, we are all salespeople at some points in our lives. We constantly are trying to get people to "pick up what we put down". When you interview for a job, you are selling the value you would bring to a company. When you ask someone on a date, you are selling them the idea that you might make a great companion. The best way to sell something is with catchy marketing. Good marketers know how to spin features to make them seem catchy while shady marketers may simply lie in a catchy way. The most common trend are the opportunistic marketers who simply bend the truth *just* enough to be catchy, but not be *technically* a lie. They may make a quick buck, but their reputation will eventually catch up with them. When a good marketer gives exactly what was advertised, they tend to build up a good reputation and following, and ever so rarely there is something that surpasses all expectations, creating huge demand and buzz. This really raises the tide for all involved and allows others to vamp on such good will and create similar, maybe even better products. This process moves innovation forward in society. Unfortunately, anything that creates buzz attracts those opportunistic and sometimes shady marketers that can try to ride the buzz to make a quick buck. And boy has the idea of the skin microbiome created a buzz in the skincare community!

We will be the first to say that it is exciting to see how much attention the skin microbiome is currently getting. And the attention is not just within the medical community but also in commercials that tout skin products that claim to be microbiome-friendly or microbiome-gentle (as discussed in Chapter 5). The number of skin care products that claim to be probiotic grows daily, as do products claiming to contain prebiotics, postbiotics, synbiotics, and more. As more research is published about the skin microbiome's involvement in disease and health and how we might modulate it to alter the skin's overall health, scientists, physicians, and skin care companies are pursuing the use of prebiotics, probiotics, and postbiotics to treat disease as well as promote the skin's health and beauty. This is wonderful since we are seeing hints of the Holobiont Philosophy in the skin care arena.

But here's the problem. While countless companies are now attempting to cash in on the microbiome craze and find ways to capitalize on the growing microbiome awareness by using terms such as probiotic and microbiome-friendly, they are using these terms very loosely and changing the way they formulate their products very little. We are all aware that many of the skin care fads out there can be quite gimmicky, and this is no exception. However, as we have discussed in the book thus far, skin microbes have a great potential to truly affect the skin's health and beauty. So how can we differentiate consumer clickbait from legitimate skin biome care? Don't worry, we got you!

Who's in Charge Here?

There is often a disconnect between the meaning of terms that skin scientists use and the ways brands use those terms for marketing. This is not new. Marketing professionals attempt to use terminology that resonates with the broadest possible demographic in order to sell the most products. Using scientific jargon, though often more nuanced and accurate, can often be too confusing for the layperson and thus may not resonate and lead to product sales. Because of this, marketing professionals often take a scientific principle and boil it down to a catchy phrase that may or may not be completely accurate and may or may not be reductive or oversimplified in nature. That is just how things work. Consumers like easy, bite sized morsels of knowledge. For the skin health and aesthetics industry as a whole, the main reason for doing this is the almighty dollar (sales). When it comes to our topic at hand, the skin biome, the other driver for the way skin biome-related products are marketed is due to the ambiguity that comes from a lack of regulatory guidance, especially when it comes to probiotic topicals made for the skin (legitimate or otherwise).

Encouraging bacterial growth through topical products has not been the status quo and is quite antithetical to how topicals have been formulated, made, and regulated in the past (and mostly in the present). This is why it is only recently that regulatory bodies have begun having discussions on how to go about standardizing the implementation of microbiome-related technologies. Currently there is not any broad, sweeping consensus, and thus there is a bit of a Wild West mentality with the marketing of such products. As more companies and products are brought to the market with claims that they target the microbiome, we have started to see a discrepancy in how companies are defining terms such as probiotics, which can have serious implications for how the layperson buys into a brand or product. It has become an issue, then, when companies that sell products claiming probiotic, prebiotic, and postbiotic ingredients take advantage of the ambiguity of these terms. This tactic can be problematic when there is also a general lack of understanding on what those terms mean to the consumer.

While at the time of writing this there is some legislation that may act to tighten up the regulation of cosmetic products in the United States, there are no current global regulations or guidelines that govern how cosmetic products that are intended to modulate the microbiome are governed. That is also true regarding regulatory bodies such as the FDA in the United States. Since that is the case, companies are left to self-regulate these products the same way they self-regulate all their other cosmetic products. They must thus ensure that the products they produce are safe and deliver the benefits they claim. However, if the claim is ambiguously defined, how does a consumer know if the company is delivering what it claims? For instance, there is no regulated definition for microbiome-safe, microbiome-friendly, or microbiome-gentle. While there are a couple of companies that are trying to put a stake in the ground as the authority by which these parameters should be decided, companies are left defining these terms on their own. So where does that leave the consumer? What do these products do for the consumer? If a product says it's microbiome-safe, friendly, or gentle, does that really mean it is?

There is beginning to be a little more clarity on that last question since some regulatory bodies are starting to come together on the topic of skin microbiome in cosmetics and attempting to find a way to align this. However, some of the proposed definitions can be a bit too reductive and potentially problematic. An example is the *International Cooperation on Cosmetics Regulation (ICCR)* that published in 2021 a summary report called "Microbiome and Cosmetics: Survey of Products, Ingredients, Terminologies and Regulatory Approaches." The report defines some of the terms we have been discussing.

CATEGORIES	DESCRIPTIONS
Probiotic	Live or dormant micro-organisms (e.g. Lactobacillus casei, Lactobacillus acidophilus, Nitrosominas eutropha, etc.
Paraprobiotic	Non-viable probiotic cells (intact or broken) or their crude cell extracts.
Prebiotic	Nutrients for probiotics or natural skin microbiota e.g. niacinamide, minerals, thermal water, vitamins, oligosaccharides, natural oils, etc.

CATEGORIES	DESCRIPTIONS
Postbiotic	Soluble factors (products or metabolic by-products) secreted by live bacteria or released after bacterial lysis (e.g. Bifida ferment lysate, Lactococcus ferment lysate, Bacillus coagulans ferment, etc.)
Microbiome friendly (or microbiota friendly)	Does not interfere with the skin microbiome
Other	Not captured by the above groupings (e.g. microbiome-activated, or activated by skin microbiome)

Source: Report for the International Cooperation on Cosmetics Regulation Microbiome and Cosmetics: Survey of Products, Ingredients, Terminologies and Regulatory Approaches"

While these definitions are not necessarily enforced as the current standard definitions used by marketers in the skin care industry, it is at least a start at attempting to bring some sort of standardization by which companies can be held accountable. It should be noted, however, that while the definition they aspire to for "probiotic" does not meet the scientific definition as outlined by Montalban-Arques and colleagues or the WHO (see Chapter 5), it does at least require that the microbe be considered living in order to carry the moniker of probiotic. That is a relatively low threshold to meet given the robust set of standards outlined by Montalban-Arques and colleagues, and the proposed definition does technically consider flesh eating bacteria a probiotic (it is a live microorganism, no?). So, the definition here is reductive and needs a bit more work to match the higher standards we have outlined. Despite this, it is quite concerning that much of the industry still makes claims that certain products are considered probiotic when they contain absolutely no live microbes.

BUCKING THE ANTIMICROBIAL STANDARD

While there have been food products that contain live microbes on the market for many years (e.g., yogurt), it is a relatively new phenomenon that skin care products are being produced that claim to contain live microbes. Until recently, it has been the status quo that topical products contain as few microbes as possible—the fewer the better—and thus the preservative systems that most of them use to keep microbes from growing in the product. However, this is changing. As we are learning about the need for a healthy skin microbiome, we now have a number of companies that are developing topical products specifically formulated to deliver microbes to the skin or create an environment on the skin conducive for those microbes. Although relatively few, some of these products are already on the market (e.g., BIOJUVE).

Currently, almost all (if not all) topical products that intentionally contain microbes are categorized as cosmetic products. That is intentional since cosmetic products have relatively low regulatory hurdles compared to therapeutic products. Although we can deduce that modulating the skin microbiome for the better would likely have therapeutic applications, making such a claim would require a product to be regulated as a biologic or a drug rather than a cosmetic. That would result in significant costs both in time and money for the companies that are developing these products. Companies are opting to rein back the beneficial claims they promote for these products in order to maintain their cosmetic regulatory status. That is not a bad thing as long as a company respects the consumer by using realistic and factual marketing claims regarding any microbiome-related ingredient.

While being regulated as a cosmetic has its advantages, it does not mean a company is free to develop a product any way it wants. When it comes to microbes in topical skin products, there are different sets of regulations from country to country that specify how products must be checked to be free from contaminating microbes. All these regulations are designed to prevent contamination of topical products from microbes that could potentially hurt the consumer if they find their way into a product during or after the manufacturing process. This is because most cosmetic products sit in a room temperature warehouse for many months before a consumer buys them. That allows time for even a single microbe to completely colonize a cosmetic product should it find that product a suitable environment. Regulatory bodies in each country have thus developed a set of standards to guide these product manufacturers. But these regulations are not made with topical that *intend* to deliver microbes in mind.

An example of this is in the United States where the FDA mandates that any topical be considered adulterated (and therefore not allowed on the market) if the microbes are found to be "beyond acceptable limits" as outlined in the *Bacteriological Analytical Manual* (BAM). Here is what that manual states:

> "Cosmetic products are not expected to be aseptic; however, they must be completely free of high-virulence microbial pathogens, and the total number of aerobic microorganisms per gram must be low. Since there are no widely acceptable standards for numbers, temporary guidelines are used instead. For eye-area products, counts should not be greater than 500 colony forming units (CFU)/g; for non-eye-area products, counts should not be greater than 1000 CFU/g."

Likewise, Canada sets limits as dictated by the International Standards Organization (ISO) Standards on Cosmetics-Microbiology-Microbiological Limits (ISO 17516:2014.8).

As a final example, Japan uses its "Standards for Cosmetics," which states:

"Ingredients of cosmetics, including any impurities contained therein, shall not contain anything that may cause infection or that otherwise makes the use of the cosmetic a potential health hazard."

In addition to these three examples of regulations for cosmetics, there is also a similar thread that intends to limit the amount of *pathogenic* microbes that may cause issues for the consumer if applied topically. The BAM and ISO standards above are interesting since they specifically call out any aerobic (requires oxygen to grow) microbes, whether deemed pathogenic or not. However, there are bacteria that can be either aerobic or anaerobic (do not require oxygen to grow), depending on the conditions. That makes these regulations ambiguous when it comes to microbes that may not fit into the categories listed. For instance, our favorite skin microbe, *C. acnes*, is not listed and is not aerobic. Therefore, *C. acnes* is not considered a contaminant based on these standards and could be used as a cosmetic ingredient. On the other hand, live Lactobacillus species that can be aerobic are currently used in a few product lines in the European Union where the ISO standard prohibits more than 1,000 aerobic mesophilic (grows in moderate temperatures) microbes per gram of product. So, there must be some flexibility with regulatory bodies concerning products that intend to deliver microbes, even if the microbes might cause the product to violate a current standard.

Regardless of the standards, all regulatory bodies tend to agree that consumer topical products need to be safe for consumers. Additionally, most regulatory bodies insist that any claims that are made as to the efficacy of a product be substantiated in some capacity. In some regions such as the United Kingdom, the enforcement of claim substantiation is quite robust, but unfortunately, that is not the case everywhere. Even in the United States where claim substantiation is required, there is a disappointingly low level of enforcement due to the lack of resources for cosmetic enforcement at the FDA. However, because most of the claims that a true probiotic would make (i.e., balances the microbiome, reduces inflammation, etc.) would be considered drug claims by the FDA, we don't expect companies to make such claims on cosmetic products. That makes it difficult to weed out the products where the probiotic ingredient is effective on the skin and from those that are simply gimmicks.

As we mentioned before, there is an emerging trend for everyday skin products to claim some sort of microbiome-friendly or microbiome-gentle designation. They are basically talking about how those products do or do not interfere with the balance of the microbiome. However, products that call themselves microbiome-friendly, safe, or gentle by insinuation do not actively affect the skin microbiome composition to make it worse but do not necessarily make it better either as by those claims you are insinuating that the microbiome would not be altered. Perhaps a better claim would be "promotes a healthy microbiome" or "does not contain known antimicrobial substances." Regardless, these types of designations are mainly for current products or brands that do not want to be adversely affected by the current interest in the skin biome. A similar trend is the emergence of products that claim to interact directly with or use elements of the microbiome itself in order to make the skin-microbiome interaction better, healthier, and more balanced. Here is what we should be asking: Will these claims be substantiated so we know they are accurate, and will they be allowed by the powers that be? Does anyone know what exactly makes a healthy skin microbiome universally? Time will tell.

Product development is a complex process. When it comes to any given product, whether prescription or over the counter, there are two main elements—the active ingredients and the vehicle. You may see products that on paper look the same because they have the same active ingredients, even in the same concentrations, but the environment (the supporting ingredients) makes all the difference in how the actives are absorbed into the skin, the level of irritancy, and what we call cosmetic elegance, or what makes you look forward to using the product. Even the way the product is made and the order and manner in which the products are mixed in the production process can impact the way they work on your skin. Don't get us wrong, ingredients are important, but it is also how much of each ingredient and how they interact with other ingredients that make all the difference. A preservative alone can be very friendly to skin microbes at one effective level but raise that level even a little and it can kill everything it touches. To put it in food terms, think of a recipe. Just because two chefs use the same ingredients does not mean the quality of the dish will be the same. Perhaps one makes a dish too salty, or not spicy enough. And adding the right ingredients, in the right order, at the right time can make or break a Beurre Blanc sauce! A chef who makes a cake with the same ingredients we have at home can produce a cake with a look and flavor that are very different. Thus, it won't ever be as simple as looking at the ingredients list on a topical, because they don't list how much of those ingredients are in there or how they are made.

Bastardized Terms

When it comes to skin care, what are some of the clickbait tactics we should be aware of? As we discussed in Chapter 4, there are quite a few companies that have launched products claiming to have probiotics when the formulas do not contain live microbes. For some products, this is intentional. As some companies realized that a preservative system that is easy to work may kill any microbes they would put in their products, they kill them proactively or simply use a postbiotic and call it a probiotic, assuming the consumer doesn't know the difference and won't care as long as the product delivers on some beauty claim (e.g., it is a good moisturizer). Many companies use the term *probiotic* on their products as clickbait to sell you something that may already be a great product, but just has very little differentiation for other great products. While the competition in the skin care arena is brutal, to say the least, these clickbait tactics not only make a brand look bad but also muddy the waters for true innovations with microbiome technologies that could actually move the needle in taking skin biome care to the next level. This trend of mis-using terms may soon shift, however, since some major companies have been called out for using them as clickbait.

In one recent lawsuit against a large, well-known company, the company was sued for claiming to sell probiotic technology when it was actually using "paraprobiotic" bacteria that were killed by heating, if we are to use the terminology we outlined above from the ICCR report. While we can debate on whether this practice was deceitful, given that they are far from the only company to do this (even now at the writing of this book), it was indeed clickbait. We could argue that using the term was unnecessary since even "killed" bacteria can at times have an effect on the skin. Of course, the strain of the dead microbe and whether the cell is intact or not are also important. But here is the point. If we can convince consumers to put live microbes on their faces to receive a benefit, can we not also convince them to put dead ones on? It might be easier to convince the public to do that. But one thing we do know is that many consumers (unlike you reading this book) are not willing to do much work when it comes to understanding the products they buy. They simply depend on the media to tell them what to use. And that is exactly why marketers will call something probiotic when it is not. People know that term and don't know the word paraprobiotic—yet.

The good news is that this lawsuit has discouraged some companies from following suit. A number of products currently hitting the market that may have once claimed the probiotic moniker are now embracing prebiotic and postbiotic monikers. This is certainly progress from a consumer's standpoint, and there is much less clickbait—or is there? Is the clickbait just shifting? Companies are now using the terms *prebiotics* and *postbiotics* as surrogates for probiotics. And as we saw in Chapter 4, this, too, can be a problem.

What Is a Holobiont Philosopher to Do?

How do we avoid using products that are clickbait? The answer is that you may *not* need to avoid the products. What you do need to avoid is *overpaying* for them simply because they claim to use microbiome-related technologies when the product does not contain them. As we have already seen, many of the products that claim microbiome-related technologies have some degree of efficacy due to other ingredients in the products. The companies that make them are simply trying to outcompete in a glut of skin care by claiming the latest and greatest topic in skin science—and we believe that is indeed the skin biome. But you are savvy consumers, and now we all know the difference between clickbait and what may be the real deal when we see it.

While we may not need to avoid clickbait if the product is reasonably priced, we do need to realize that most products are traditionally formulated and include harsh preservative systems and antimicrobial ingredients that do not always mesh with the Holobiont Philosophy. While you do not need to be afraid of your favorite skin care products or brands, you should make sure you do not fall prey to overpaying for a gimmicky probiotic skin care system. As the regulations and laws catch up, it will eventually be clearer which products are legitimate. For now, follow the Holobiont Philosophy (and suggestions outlined later in the book) when you're looking for topical products, and then you (and your microbes) should be good to go.

PART III
REBOOTING THE BIOME

CHAPTER 7

THE BIOMECARE REALITY

It is difficult to say what is impossible, for the dream of yesterday is the hope of today and the reality of tomorrow.
— Robert H. Goddard

The world's dirtiest man recently died after his first bath in sixty years. Amou Haji lived in the village of Dezh Gah in Iran and avoided bathing for sixty years for fear it would make him sick. A 2013 documentary called *The Strange Life of Amou Haji* chronicled his life. Not long after he was pressured to bathe in 2022, he fell ill and passed away. He was 94 years old. A decades-long bathing boycott is not what we're advocating, but we do think that it is imperative that we share with you how your skin does self-cleanse more than you may realize and that might make you rethink a few of the hygiene habits that you have.

Dr. Day: I can often spot a new mom immediately just by looking at her hands. Jane, a young woman in her early thirties, came in for an evaluation of a very itchy and painful rash on her hands. She was a new mom and told me that she was very concerned about germs making her baby ill. She washed her hands many, many times a day and used super-hot water and hand sanitizers between washings. Understandably, she wanted to give her child the best health possible and did everything she could to clean all surfaces and anything the baby may come in contact with.

Upon examination, I observed that her hands were very red, and the skin was severely irritated, raw, and virtually worn away from so much aggressive washing. It looked tight and painful. I could see lots of scaling and clear fissures (breaks) in the skin. These changes were signs that the skin was now no longer healthy and intact and was therefore more prone to infection. All her efforts were backfiring—and the worse it got, the more she washed, thinking it would help.

I explained to her that the skin has its own unique and personal immune system as well as a microbiome, a host of good microorganisms, including bacteria, that help protect her from the outside world. Just as she didn't have to think about every beat of her heart in order to stay alive, she didn't have to overwash her hands to protect them against infection. Her skin would naturally do it for her. The more she interfered with that effort, the less protected she was from potential harm. Proper hand washing is important and necessary, but as with anything, too much of a good thing leads to trouble.

SKIN CARE IS ONLY *PART* OF BIOMECARE

We believe in staying a "little dirty." Not dirty as in literal dirt, like Amou Haji, but dirty as in not overly cleaning and exfoliating so you can retain some of your inimitable scents and oils *you* make as well as your skin's resident microbes, and the scents and substances *they* make.

Not only was your skin designed to handle exposure to the outside world, including legitimately dirty things such as pollutants and harmful microbes; but it thrives when you help maintain its ecosystem. No matter how much you wash your skin or pour on hand sanitizer, any microbes you wash away or kill will almost instantly either return or be replaced by another one that you may not want. Microbes are like those little sand crabs you see at the beach. They burrow into the sand, leaving behind a hole. Then the waves arrive and wash over them, and once the waves recede, all the sand crabs pop up again. It's the same with trying to rid ourselves of microbes. They'll always be there and pop back up. Some may be helpful, some may be harmful, and some may be neutral, but there's no way to externally eradicate them, even if we want to. Remember, humans have tried and failed at the idea of a germ-free human.

Can You Get Too Clean?

Western society is obsessed with the word *clean*—and not just clean, but *squeaky* clean. You can blame that on soap manufacturers that planted those ads in magazines and on TV decades ago. This must-be-clean notion continues to get worse with antibacterial agents included in countless products being sold to consumers on the premise that sterile equals good or safe. Sterile *is* good in the operating room or when referring to medical equipment such as syringes—anytime you're going beyond the skin and into the body—but not when it comes to the skin. Although we as a society should have learned by now about the false sentiment that cleaner is better, we have not, and it has become a real problem.

Precautions against pathogens should not dictate what's healthy for our skin and how we should care for it every day—even during something unusually risky like a pandemic. A squirt of hand sanitizer might be called for when trying to avoid spreading any contagions, and appropriate hand washing is wise, but using sanitizer or washing your hands with soap every time you touch *anything* will do more harm than good. Humans don't live in a sterile world. Everything we come in contact with is covered with microbes. Even an operating room that has been sanitized will eventually find itself covered in microbes despite the best efforts to keep it clean.

Our biology allows us to develop a commensal—sometimes symbiotic—relationship with our microbiomes that not only helps train our immune system to live in a microbe-ridden world but also helps the body avoid picking up pathogenic microbes. So we must be conscious about disrupting the balance of our skin's microbiome. Dysbiosis can affect our skin's ability to fend off unwanted microbes that constantly bombard us. In addition to environmental contagions, some microbes that already live on our skin and in our gut are opportunists, and if we get rid of our balanced microbiome by oversterilizing our skin or overusing antibiotics, a small number of these opportunists can sometimes survive the attempts to wipe them out. If so, they can take over before our good bacteria can catch up, and results are potentially life-threatening infections.

The fact is you *can* be too clean. Overcleansing can not only rid your skin of the essential, oil-rich ecosystem that houses your balanced microbiome but can also create an environment that is conducive to fostering pathogenic microbes. Of course, that doesn't mean you don't need to clean your skin at all, but it does mean that it's not healthy to be obsessed with the process. It also means we should be a bit more picky about the products we use to cleanse our skin.

To an extent, your skin is naturally self-cleaning, with new skin cells constantly rising to the surface, sweat washing over it, and new oils pushing out the contents of the pores and follicles. All the things your skin pushes to the surface create an ecosystem, an environment that is designed to protect you because they're meant to shield your skin from everyday environmental stressors. When you try to get too clean, here is what happens:

- You strip away the oils, salts, and stratum corneum—and with it the ecosystem and environment that fosters your skin's ability to defend itself.

- You remove not only some of the healthy microbiome but also the food sources for some key helpful microbes.

- When you remove the oil and microbiome-rich stratum corneum, you are removing the outermost layer that holds in moisture and protects you from UV rays and external insults such as pollutants and pathogens and can lead to irritation of the underlying skin. Without that moisture, the skin reacts by overproducing some of what was just removed. That can result in issues such as oily skin and scalp, itchiness, dryness, and flaking.

It can make your skin peel unevenly. It can make some skin cells exfoliate faster than others, which will leave your skin red, itchy, uncomfortable, and more prone to infection because the micro-breaks are exposing your skin to the elements and more potentially pathogenic microbes.

- On your skin, oil is worth its weight in gold. Less oil can lead to a reduction in the microbes that produce antioxidants and anti-microbial peptides that are specific to pathogens. It can also indirectly raise skin pH and create a more suitable environment for dangerous microbes such as pathogenic strains of *Staphylococcus aureus*. Growth of these types of microbes leaves the skin vulnerable to diseases such as dermatitis and staph infections.

Reduced antioxidants, raised pH, irritation from pathogenic microbes, overproduction of oil that is constantly being washed away—that is what can happen when we wash our skin too much, and it is a recipe for disaster.

Dr. Day: I have patients who come in with acne or breakouts, and I ask them about their cleansing routine. They often confess that they use alcohol wipes or hydrogen peroxide on their skin to dry it out and try to kill the bacteria that causes acne. I gently tell them that those chemicals are particularly toxic to their skin and actually have no effect on the bacteria they have been told causes acne. Unwittingly, they've hurt their skin, left it parched, and likely made their acne worse. (We'll discuss this at length in the next chapter, but you should know for now that acne skin does not equal dirty skin.)

Overcleansing can also cause a loss of radiance. What makes skin look dull is when skin cells pile up unevenly. If your skin is a smooth, even plane, the light that hits your face synchronously reflects off of it, and its smoothness is pleasing to the eye. On the other hand, skin that's unhealthy and has either some dryness or flakes (even micro-flakes) will bend the light as it passes through, reflecting it at different angles. That skin is not going to look radiant and clear but rather dull and older than its years.

When your skin is healthy, it goes through a normal cycle of renewal where it clears out any damaged cells and damaged extracellular matrix (e.g., damaged collagen or elastin) and replaces it with new, fresh tissue. But when your skin microbiome is out of balance and unhealthy, inflamed, and disrupted, your skin, instead of focusing on renewal, has to spend precious resources to attempt to bring the skin microflora environment back into balance. It also has to try to clear the damage done by free radicals or other environmental insults that are now getting through since the first-defense barrier may have been stripped away. It's kind of like an ant hill; disrupt it, and the ants have to rebuild it instead of gathering the food they need and staying hidden from predators.

Selling the Suds

As you learned in Chapter 6, consumers are bombarded with ads with allegedly truthful information about the skin care products they need. One of the most egregious exaggerations is that you need a lot of lather, whether from soap or shampoos, in order to get truly clean.

One of the more common lathering agents in cleansing products is a chemical called sodium lauryl sulfate. It's a foaming agent and surfactant that's horrible for your skin because it breaks up the natural barrier as it washes away your skin's oils. As you know by now, these oils are critical not only for properly sealing the skin but also as the food source for the good bacteria and keeping the bad bacteria (e.g., certain strains of *S. aureus*) away. It's inexpensive and lathers well, and we have been trained to equate more lather with getting cleaner. It also changes the environment of your skin, which spells potentially bad news for the skin microbiome, depending on how often your wash, what other ingredients are in the cleanser, and what products you use after you wash.

Skin care companies found that when they removed these foaming agents, the lather wasn't as robust. When they did consumer testing, they discovered that consumers thought the soap wasn't working if it wasn't lathering. Rather than taking the time and risk failing at educating consumers, these companies decided to keep the lathering components in the products. To this day, most people use cleansers with too much surfactant and foaming agents since that is what we expect of a "good soap." Many people with skin issues may not know that the use of these products—the ones they believe are keeping them very clean—are actually contributing to their irritated skin. For example, many people with eczema who stop using their body washes on their arms and legs often see their eczema improve without the need for medication or any other treatment. Even if you don't have eczema, you still want to avoid any products with sodium lauryl sulfate and other harsh surfactants to help keep your skin as healthy as possible.

Overcleansing Makes You Dirty

As we've discussed, overcleansing can lead to changes to your skin's environment. It can change which microbes grow in which locations. It can change how many there are, and some of them may not be so good for you. And *now* you're dirty!

This goes back to the definition of what a germ is (see Chapter 1). You may think you're dirty if you have *any* bacteria on you, but overcleansing to get rid of them can produce more of the *wrong* types of bacteria. Once you stop thinking that all germs are bad, you can stop being afraid of the bacteria you actually need—this will allow you to safely and appropriately cleanse your skin and still make it look its best.

Dr. Hitchcock: When I was approaching puberty, I had perfect skin (save a chicken pox scar or two). However, I noticed that my sister who was a couple years older began using an apricot scrub that everybody seemed to have (but shouldn't have) in those days. I was jealous because my parents were buying her a lot of products, and all they gave me was a bar of soap. After begging my stepmother, who advised me not to mess with my skin if I didn't need to, I was finally allowed to get my first skin care product, a witch hazel astringent. A day or so after I started using it, my skin began to dry out, which soon led to my skin breaking out. My skin had been flawless until I started messing with it. I'm sure my burgeoning hormones may have been a factor, but disrupting my skin's natural balance didn't help. I fought acne for several years with witch hazel instead of trying the simplest of all strategies—leaving my skin alone.

The Best Way to Wash

The best way to wash your face and body is basically a nice rinse with just water. You can use a gentle cleanser and water if you must, but water alone will rinse most of what you need to wash away. When it comes to exfoliation, drying your face with a towel will help remove some of the outer layer of stratum corneum that is ready to come off and blot some excess oils. Just make sure you change and wash your towels regularly.

Any area with hair or places you sweat a lot (e.g., genitals and underarms) probably could use soap due to the apocrine sweat gland secretions in those areas as well as the moist nature of the skin in those places. These moist areas are a haven for growth of certain microbes that can turn your apocrine sweat into body malodor (more on this later). So you might want to routinely use a gentle soap or cleanser there, although it is not essential if you are able to deal with a little bit of musky smell (most of us in the United States are not as tolerant of that as other parts of the world).

Those who wear makeup should always remove it at night because makeup left on your skin can be toxic to your microbiome and your skin since it attracts and holds onto pollution. That pollution left on your skin decomposes to elements that can be harmful, increases discoloration, and can even lead to skin cancer if chronically left unchecked. Water might be fine for removing some of the makeup and pollution if you use something special like a microfiber cloth that will remove most of the makeup without any assistance from soap or cleansers. We are not kidding. Try it. You can also use micellar water or a gentle cleanser to get those hard-to-remove makeup products (e.g., eyeliner and mascara).

Dr. Day: If you're happy with the condition of your skin, that's fabulous. Keep using what you're using. There's no need to mess with it. I see patients every day who come in with a full bag of products, and they tell me they're using all of them, and nothing works. Their skin is breaking out and irritated. It has an uneven tone and looks old. I tell them, "Okay, then let's try nothing for a bit." I have them stop using all products, rinse only with micellar water, use no soap, and not rub their skin for a week. Sometimes using nothing works perfectly.

Once their skin has recovered from using the wrong products, we slowly start adding back select products, one or two at a time, that I select for their skin rather than layering five or more at once. We are now able to get their skin to a healthy radiance, restore their biome, and appropriately address their skin needs.

Odor is *not* a four-letter word

We all have a unique odor caused by our genetics, the substances our cells produce and secrete, and our microbiome and what they secrete. It's why perfume never smells the same on everyone and why you might react viscerally to someone whose natural scent you find off-putting, often for no discernible reason. We hope you don't consider your own scent a negative but as something to cherish about yourself.

Dr. Day: One of my strongest memories is a conversation I had with my sister when she was battling cancer. About a month before she died, she told me that she no longer smelled like herself. She said she didn't smell like anything at all, and I could see how that scared her. I had never thought much about odor, and when I did it was mostly about how to cover it up. It never occurred to me that we each have a unique smell and that we can lose it. Throughout my education and practice in dermatology, smell has been an important component of my understanding of illness and health. Patients with psoriasis flares smell like keratin, the protein that makes up most of the skin. Patients who are ill often have an unusual odor. Cysts have a common pungent odor when we drain them. So much of what I do relies on using all my senses to understand and help my patients.

It is not your unique body's natural scent that is ever the issue. It is malodor (*mal* means bad) caused by specific interactions in the skin biome that most people want to avoid. Body scent can change based on diet and activity. Another change can take place when we try to sterilize certain areas, especially the underarms. That causes a shift in the types of microbes, including fungus and bacteria, that proliferate there as well as the substances our bodies produce (similar to how oil production changes when we overwash our face). When certain species of bacteria proliferate and eat certain body secretions, the molecules they produce can change your body's normal scent to body malodor.

People tend to smell more when they exercise because their sweat is more abundant. This provides the microbes on certain areas of the skin with an abundance of a food source which when metabolized by the microbes turns into odiferous substances such as certain fatty acids, steroids, and sulfur compounds—all smelly types of molecules. What you're smelling are the by-products of an intricate interaction of the secretions of certain skin glands with the microbes that tend to reside in those areas. Your body doesn't produce such malodor on its own. And because the types of bodily secretions and microbes that live in certain areas tend to be common in any given population, when we do have body odor—the underarm tang or the reek emanating from your teen's shoes—it will typically smell similar no matter who has it. Slight variations in body odor can happen due to gender, age, and a variation in diet. While some body odor is normal, it is the really offensive odors you want to get rid of, and they're often exacerbated when your microbiome is out of balance.

Researchers at Dr. Hitchcock's company are looking at whether it might be possible to negate body odor through the use of microbes or micro-metabolites, but until that happens, relish your individual scent. Don't overwash yourself because that will contribute to dysbiosis that can enhance body malodor. If you do choose to use deodorant, make sure you are picky about the ingredients, and avoid harsh or irritating ones. If you like, enhance your unique scent with perfume or cologne to bring out certain flavors of your own uniqueness rather than eliminate them. But never be afraid to live a fragrance-free life, because sometimes just smelling like a clean and healthy human is the best scent money can buy. If you've ever inhaled the delicious scent of a baby's little head, you know what we mean.

Skin Detox: Not a Thing

You do not need to detoxify your skin. What does that even mean? Skin detox is a category of something that doesn't actually exist. It's a gimmick created by certain companies to sell you more products you don't need. You won't be getting any unique benefits from overnight detox creams and oils, charcoal masks, or natural clay body washes. Don't fall for the hype.

Your *skin's* job is to detoxify itself. That's what the liver is for. What other toxicity are we talking about? It's just imaginary toxicity—and trying to get rid of it can be destructive to your natural skin microbiome and thus your skin biome. As we feel there is little to this topic, we won't go on. However, we did want to address it as the associated buzzwords do tend to separate quite a few people from their hard-earned dollars, all while messing with the skin biome.

Hand Sanitizer: A Great Tool That Is Overused

Hand sanitizers are quite misunderstood. There is a place and a reason for hand sanitizers. They're great tools for those who work in places such as hospitals that are at high risk for microbial pathogens. Protective gear such as nitrile gloves, masks, and scrubs also allow healthcare workers to go from patient to patient quickly while lowering their risk of spreading any microbial pathogens among them.

That doesn't mean hand sanitizers are necessary or healthy for you to use every day and especially not all hours of the day. In 2020, fear of viral pathogens led to bottles of hand sanitizer flying off the shelves and manufacturers scrambling to meet the demand. Then came the wave of unsafe alternatives since people were desperate for a stash of the stuff and thought they could simply read the label on the hand sanitizer bottle and use the same ingredients to make their own or follow the advice on Internet DIY videos that were usually incorrect.

What most people didn't know is the actual science behind the manufacture of hand sanitizers. They didn't realize that adding certain ingredients can ruin the utility of the formula or that certain alcohols contain poisonous methanol. They didn't know that increasing the alcohol concentration doesn't necessarily make the product more effective. Often the higher alcohol levels made the sanitizer *less* effective.

The widespread and chronic use of hand sanitizers can also wreak havoc on your skin, its microbiome, and its innate immune system. Frequent use can lead to dry, cracked skin that makes it easier for pathogens or infections to get in. It also greatly reduces the normal exposure of your immune system to the everyday "dirt" that our hands introduce to the rest of the skin and the mouth. That can change the way your body reacts to the same microbes it normally doesn't care about. It weakens the immune system, which makes you more likely to have an inflammatory response or be susceptible to pathogens.

In addition, constantly putting antimicrobial substances on your skin can result in fostering the emergence of microbes that are resistant to those antimicrobials, making them less effective. We've seen this with antibiotics. For most people, simply washing your hands with soap and water when appropriate is enough to keep you safe and healthy, and it reduces the potential downsides of habitual use of a product that's not intended for chronic use. This is an example of a good tool being used incorrectly. However, when common sense prevails, it can be a great addition to the health of those that need it when used appropriately.

THE BIOMECARE MINIMILIST

Skin biomecare is so much better for your skin than the skin care products you've been using all your life. Even the best products can't yet replicate 100% of what your body produces when healthy. The problem is that Skin biomecare is not yet a mainstream idea, so finding the right products can be tricky (there are many gimmicks out there).

No one needs to use a lot of different products. As we said in the previous section, water and maybe a gentle cleanser, microfiber cloth or micellar water are enough for cleansing. A good, simple moisturizer is enough for hydration, and some people may not even need a moisturizer at certain times. You do not need a *lot* of serums, toners, and expensive potions. The operative word here being *a lot*. With skin biome care, less is more.

Dr. Day: There are many serums I like and recommend daily to support skin repair and anti-aging functions without hurting the microbiome, and they can be layered. But you don't need an eighteen-step daily routine for beautiful skin. I like eye products for the eye area because that is the thinnest skin on the body and can be more sensitive than other parts of the face. It's also very important to pat, not rub, the product into your skin during application to avoid any stretching and irritation and to improve penetration of the products into the skin.

And keep in mind that some of those lotions and potions you love may be okay to use. For instance, adding a vitamin C serum to your face is a great (although short-lived) antioxidant that helps your body fight free radicals. When looking for these serums, simple is often better. Both in the number of products used, as well as the number of ingredients in each product.

Dr. Hitchcock: After giving a lecture on post-procedure skin care, one of the attendees came up and told me she had such bad rosacea that she had to use an assortment of topicals, prescription meds and a heavy concealer, and she wondered if I had any advice as to why she still had a lot of inflammation. I asked her what she was using on her skin, and she listed eleven products she used every day. I challenged her to go back to her dermatologist and see if she could be weaned off some of them, and then to try a month or two where all she used was a bland moisturizer and a gentle cleanser. She did. And she contacted me soon after to report that her rosacea was now a thing of the past.

Biome-Friendly Formulation: Ingredients Primer

The Most Effective Ingredients

Most skin care companies are aware of two things most people do when they get a new product. First, they smell it. Next, they put it on the back of their hand to see how it feels. Many products might smell wonderful and feel even better, **but neither of these things are indicators of how good the product is for your skin**, let alone your skin biome as a whole. There are many ingredients that are routinely used in quality skin care and a few ingredient types that are staples in skin care (retinoids, antioxidants, moisturizing agents). However, to date, very little has been done to determine how these ingredients alone or in formulation affect the skin microbiome—for better or for worse. So, if an ingredient is great for the skin cells but causes disruption of the skin microbiome, which in turn is then bad for the skin biome, would you still consider it great for the skin?

The good news is that we are discovering that some of the ingredients we love don't adversely affect the microbiome and may even help it. Ingredients such as colloidal oatmeal have been studied for how they might affect the skin microbiome in people who have atopic dermatitis. In a study by Johnson & Johnson, it was found that "treatment with the 1% colloidal oat eczema cream was associated with trends towards lower prevalence of Staphylococcus species and higher microbiome diversity at lesion sites."[1] While diversity isn't always associated with microbiome health of the skin, in areas such as the forearm where eczema can be prevalent, this type of diversity is associated with healthy skin. Additionally, from Dr. Hitchcock's labs at Crown Laboratories we have research that has investigated how retinoids can affect the integrity of the skin microbiome. Interestingly, some retinoids such as retinol and retinyl palmitate have very little if any effect on a critical component of the facial skin microbiome, *C. acnes*, while other retinoid type molecules such as bakuchiol and hydroxypinacolone retinoate (HPR) have a highly antimicrobial effect on it. We are starting to see that in the future we will need to curate which ingredients, and what amounts of those ingredients, are appropriate for skin biomecare versus simply skin care alone.

As mentioned in Chapter 6, the claims microbiome-gentle, microbiome-friendly, and other similar claims have recently appeared on some skin product labels. To date, there is no industry regulation on what these terms mean and what methods or standards should be used to allow companies to make such claims for their products. After all, we are still wrapping our heads around the science of the skin microbiome and still learning what it truly means to have a healthy microbiome. So if a company claims that its products are microbiome-friendly or microbiome-gentle, what does that mean? How did the company test those products? There are some organizations and companies that are trying to set the standards for the industry by selling their tests and provide their "stamp of approval" to make these claims. However, more transparency and collaboration is needed before consumers know what it means to buy products that make these claims. For now, take these types of claims with a grain of salt, and simply look at the product label to see if the ingredients seem to agree with such a claim.

THE BASIC PREBIOTIC/PROBIOTIC/POSTBIOTIC BIOMECARE REGIMEN

With all the unknowns regarding which products are good for the skin alone versus the skin and the microbiome, how do we know how to choose what is best for our biomes? As we know more, we can do better. But for now, we'll make some suggestions based on what is known about the skin and its microbiome. Keep in mind that as science evolves, so will our skin biomecare recommendations. This basic regimen, however, will work for most people with normal, healthy skin. (We'll cover some specific issues in the next chapter.)

The regimen is divided into two parts: (1) for the face and (2) for specific areas of your body. For optimal results, you should use unique products for each one because the microbiome of each area is completely different.

For the face, follow these steps:

Morning Must Haves:

- Wash or rinse your face with water. If necessary, include a gentle cleanser with little surfactant to avoid drying out the skin and removing your microbes and all the great skin-healthy substances they produced during the night. Remember, your skin oils and secretions are the best *prebiotics* for your skin microbiome, so try to retain as much of them as possible when cleansing.

- Apply sun protection. While UV protection is always a good idea, some sunscreen ingredients, while highly effective at blocking UV rays, can be antimicrobial. An example of this is zinc oxide, a wonderful active that has been used successfully for many years to block UV rays, but it is an antimicrobial when used alone. The question is whether or not applying a zinc oxide sunscreen on bare skin will adversely affect the biome. If you overcleanse and there is little of the oil barrier to keep the zinc oxide from the microbes, then the answer is yes, it will probably cause disruption. However, if you use only water to cleanse your face in the morning or use a cleanser that allows you to retain your oils, then using zinc oxide should be okay. Additionally, if the zinc oxide is coated with specific substances, it can retain all its UV protectiveness while not bothering the microbiome. A final way to seal in those microbes to protect them from any topicals you may put on that can affect them is to use the right moisturizer, which can have ingredients that provide a barrier between the skin biome and other products such as makeup and sunscreens. We will discuss that soon.

Morning Nice to Haves:

- Serums are popular and quite frankly wonderful to use. However, that is true only if the serum contains the right active ingredients. As we already mentioned, choosing serums with the right actives can be great for biomecare. However, serums with antimicrobial actives may cause disruption if you use them every day. One great thing to look for in a serum is a film-forming agent to protect the skin biome. While that might sound occlusive, you won't even know the film is there since these film formers are breathable in most cases and can act to protect your microbiome from other topicals such as makeup that you might put on your face before leaving your home.

- Moisturize as needed. That is something most people misunderstand. Not everyone needs to use a moisturizer all the time. Your skin's oils should do most of the moisturizing, but as we age and during the winter months, we might need some assistance. A simple, no-nonsense moisturizer should suffice. Keep in mind that the more fancy ingredients there are in a moisturizer, the more potential it has to mess with your microbiome. So, keep it simple. Just like a serum, a moisturizer with a film-forming agent is a great way to protect the microbes on the skin.

- For both serums and moisturizers, this is a great chance to introduce *postbiotics* into your regimen. These postbiotics should be from a strain of microbes that secrete skin-relevant substances (not all microbes secrete the good stuff).

Evening Must Haves:

- Wash to remove your makeup; use a gentle cleanser with skin biomecare in mind.

- Moisturize (see the Morning Nice to Haves).

Evening Nice to Haves:

- Evening is the best time to use your live *probiotic* products. As we mentioned in Chapter 6, in order for a true probiotic to work its magic, it needs time to engraft onto the skin. Putting it on your skin right before bedtime provides those wonderful little symbiotes time to work their magic for a good six, seven, or eight hours (or more) while you slumber.

- Apply retinol if you desire, but make sure the type of retinol you are using, and its formulation is not antimicrobial.

Dr. Hitchcock: Regarding legitimate skin probiotics, there is currently a dearth of them on the market. So I have developed a simple regimen of products with the Holobiont Philosophy in mind. They can be found under the brand name BIOJUVE. They include topicals that condition the skin biome to a place of symbiosis, as well as a topical with live skin-native microbes that help you curate the skinmicrobiome. The aim is to provide the skin biome with the right living strains, the right nutrients and the right environment. I am hopeful that more such products will become prevalent in the near future. These products are especially useful for those who are trying to wean themselves from too many topicals and restore their natural ecosystems —basically trying to put the grey wolves back in Yellowstone National Park.

SIDEBAR ABOUT EXFOLIATION

Mechanistically, our skin is designed to push things out. It is always creating new skin cells that rise to the surface. Our sebaceous glands are always forming new oil and pushing it to the surface. It's the same with your hair. For either our skin or our hair, all we have to do is wipe the surface, and they self-clean in a way with some assistance. At first that might sound odd, but when we distance ourselves from the error of the squeaky-clean dogma, it starts to make a lot more sense.

The microbes of your skin tend to settle in (engraft) by building little structures with what are called biofilms. When we scrape the skin or remove large amounts of the stratum corneum, it becomes like a demolition team tearing down all those microbes' homes. If the homes were filled with pathogens, that's great. But if you have healthy skin, it is likely you just tore down the homes of billions of your best friends. And guess what? Someone is going to buy that land and redevelop it into new homes, and you'd better hope it isn't someone looking to cause trouble for your skin.

Gentle exfoliation is an important step in any biome-care regimen, but because your skin cell turnover slows down with age, it's not something you need to do every day. Exfoliation should always be gentle—no harsh scrubs or strong acid exfoliants. Remember, the outer layer of skin (the stratum corneum) is home to an ecosystem that is important to your skin. While some gentle coercion to get the most outer skin cells to drop off is merited, anything more is not only unnecessary but unhealthy. Many people don't understand how much they are traumatizing their skin when their exfoliation process is too aggressive. For people who do not use makeup, exfoliation is not as essential. But for those who do use makeup, exfoliation can act to brighten the skin and allow topicals and makeup to apply flawlessly. As with most things we have discussed, balance is key.

A great exfoliator we recommend that is microbiome-compatible contains beta hydroxy acid or salicylic acid. One half to two percent salicylic acid is available in over-the-counter products and makes a great microbiome-compatible exfoliant for your biomecare regimen, and it is also a great ingredient for acne-prone skin (more on that later). But use sparingly since overuse can disrupt the skin's ecosystem just like harsh exfoliants.

An exfoliator (more like a skin terrorizer) that we do *not* recommend is anything with ground up peach pits, walnut shells, or the like. These ingredients are far too aggressive and abrasive and will scratch and damage your skin. They will also ruin the home of your outermost microbiome until your skin is able to heal. Just don't do it. Your skin will thank you.

Scalp and Hair

Shampoos are made to strip oils and excess grooming products away, so if you wash too often you will begin to leave the scalp void of natural oils and your body will respond with production of excess oils to compensate. So, unless your hair is unusually oily, there's no need to wash your hair every day. If the ends of your hair are dry, apply conditioner there only—not on your roots. Check the label on your conditioner. You might be surprised to find that it contains surfactants to help rinse out the conditioner, which is why you could also use it as a gentler shampoo.

Companies that make consumers feel they must shampoo and condition their hair during every shower or bath are savvy marketers, but trust us that doing such is not a necessity. They sell products infused with the notion of things that feel good in the moment. Yes, it *does* feel good when you wash your hair. But guess what, it's not just your hair that's been conditioned—*you* have literally been conditioned to enjoy that brand of clean. If you have been washing every day, don't worry as all you need to do is gradually add more time between washes until you are only washing once or twice a week, or as needed depending on the grooming products you use.

Nobody Likes Change, But Everybody Likes Improvement

Dr. Day: As wearing masks became the norm during around COVID-19, I started to notice that several patients a day were coming in with styes around their eyes and rashes around their mouths and noses. I quickly realized that what was happening—the microbes from the mouth were being trapped on the skin and then escaping through any gaps in connection between the mask and the skin. The microbes were forced upwards towards the eyes and then got trapped by the eyelashes along the eyelid-conjunctival borders. There they would cause redness, infection, and swelling. Increased friction and humidity around the mouth, along with the occlusion from the mask, caused skin breakdown and allowed the mouth microbes, which are not native to the skin, to penetrate and lead to infection. As with over washing, over-wearing masks too long can lead to a greater risk of infection, without a greater protection against disease. I created and patented a serum to address this issue and found that using that, along with using a mouth wash that contained 2% hydrogen peroxide, was very helpful in resolving the issues.

Nobody likes change, but change is inevitable and often forced on us at the most inconvenient times. There is no better example of this than during the COVID-19 pandemic when skin ecosystem-modifying habits became the norm, including self-isolation, mask-wearing, and overuse of soaps and sanitizers. These changes occurred suddenly and were maintained over long periods. Stories like Dr. Day's were not unusual during the pandemic. As she mentioned, these habits caused sudden and drastic changes to areas of the skin where the body did not have time to properly acclimate. That led to a lot of individuals with various skin issues induced by these changes.

This is a phenomenon that is not unique to the pandemic. Sudden changes in our skin environment happen a few times in our lives. At birth we are thrust from the safety of our mothers' womb where there is thought to be a very low level of controlled microbes to the outside world riddled with microbes of every make and model. That sudden change is what is thought to cause baby acne and similar skin issues early in life. When we hit puberty, the sebaceous glands of the skin open their floodgates, creating an all-you-can-eat buffet for microbes that had been living secluded lives deep in the follicles until then. That sudden change is why many teens have some acne during that time. When someone has a skin care regiment they follow for many years and then changes to a very different regimen, the skin often breaks out due to the change in the skin's environment.

These examples show that we should not overreact to skin issues caused by sudden changes in the skin environment. Instead, we should seek to understand whether the issue is a transient one due to that change or something more that requires medical attention and intervention. Usually, it is the former. If you attempt to follow our recommendations for the best skin biomecare, don't freak out if you notice a spot or two during the transition. If a newborn baby can get through it and end up with perfect skin using minimal products, so can you.

CHAPTER 8

NOT A FAN OF BUGS

There is but one temple in the world,
and that is the body of man.
—Novalis

Dr. Hitchcock: I am not a fan of bugs—not bugs as in the colloquialism for bacteria but as in insects. I briefly had a roommate in grad school (let's call him Jackson) who was earning his Master's degree in entomology—the study of bugs. We didn't last long as roommates. I once saw on our porch what looked like a large (very large) ant with red and black velvety fur all over its body. I had never seen anything like it before, even during my years in Cub Scouts. For me, it was the stuff of nightmares, something from a science fiction movie. It was actually what I now know to be commonly referred to as a velvet ant, which is actually not an ant at all but a type of family of wasps whose females lack wings.

"What is that?" I yelped.

"Oh, it's actually a wasp of some sort," he (way too) calmly replied.

Noting his calm demeanor, I added, "Well, I hope they don't get in our apartment, because just looking at it has my skin crawling."

I'll never forget what he said next that ended the conversation. "Yeah, and they taste terrible."

I thought he was joking but then found out that he often ate various kinds of bugs in his "quest" for all there is to know about his chosen field of study. I suppose it was admirable in a way. In the years since, I can't say that I haven't done some experimentation on myself that others might find equally unsavory (e.g., covering my face with billions of C. acnes defendens to see what happened, before it was cool).

On another occasion, I woke up early in the morning because I was freezing cold. I walked into the living room and found the front door wide open and my roommate sleeping on the floor right in front of it. Had he not been snuggled up in a sleeping bag I would have wondered if someone had broken into the apartment, murdered him, and escaped, leaving the door wide open. I woke him up and asked what was going on.

"Oh, I left the door open all night in order to help our apartment establish better equilibrium with that of nature," he muttered as he rubbed drool from his mountain-man-like beard that had been growing more and more unkempt since we moved in.

As I stood there speechless, he saw my face and added, "I slept in front of the door, so you didn't have to worry about intruders or anything."

In my head I retorted with "Intruders? You mean like all the bugs that came in whilst I slept? Like a family of those velvet ant-waspy things that, by the way, sting people?"

But I knew he was in his own world. It was not a bad world, maybe a bit eccentric, but it just was not a world I wanted to be part of. I simply asked him not to do it again, and our cohabitation ended shortly thereafter.

So yes, I would like to keep my life bug-free. However, as a scientist I do realize that bugs are an important and unavoidable part of any ecosystem. Just as I don't attempt to sterilize my body, I realize that I can't keep my home bug-free. In fact, there are thought to be on average around 100 types of bugs in any given household.[1] I just don't want to see them. I think many of us may feel that way as well, some more than others.

I understand why people react with disgust when I talk about bacteria being all over their faces. They might appreciate it, but they just don't want to talk about it. And that is just fine as long as they <u>understand</u> that their skin's an ecosystem, bugs and all, and so we need to care for it as one.

Why Bugs (Insects) and Bugs (Microbes) Shouldn't Bug Us

There are three types of people: (1) those who suck up every bug they see with the vacuum cleaner and lock that vacuum in some remote part of the house so they can forget what terror lies inside, (2) those who lovingly trap household bugs under a cup and take them outside to live free in nature, and (3) those, like Dr. Day, who could probably set new world records in sprinting as they run the other way if a bug is anywhere in sight. None of that changes the reality that those same bugs or their relatives can easily make their way back into the house, and likely they do, even the ones you may think are stuck in the vacuum. The fact is that there is no invisible barrier around our homes that keeps anything non-human out. We can use pesticides to provide a type of bug barrier, but most of the poisons we use to rid our homes of bugs are poisons to us, our children, and our pets as well.

The fact is that if a bug finds the ecosystem within our house conducive to life, it will likely move in. If it does not, it will find somewhere else to live. If a fly gets in the house, it usually flies around frantically for a bit and then dies. However, if we leave food out, it can feed on it and then lay eggs and start a family. It's the same with roaches and other bugs. The ecosystem we create in our homes dictates what organisms move in. If we clean often and well, we will have a very different ecosystem than if we never cleaned. If we never dust, then certain things will flourish than if we dust regularly. There are thought to be 9,000 species of microbes that live on household dust alone, which provides food for certain bugs that feed bigger bugs—and you get the idea.

While there are differences between the inside of your home and the outdoors, it is only something that is due to the differences in things such as climate (access to sunlight, AC, furnace, dehumidifier), food sources (food left out), and hygienic practices. Unless the home is hermetically sealed, nature will eventually take it over if you walk away from it. So the inside is *really* still the same as the outside, just with a very controlled environment that curates what exists within.

That is also true for the biomes of our bodies. We have often referred to the gut and skin biomes as separate entities (and they are), but just like the creation of an indoor space separate from the outdoors, the gut is a creation of space separate from the outside. From the study of embryology, the science of how an organism develops from germ cells (sperm, egg) into a functional human being, we know that in the very early stages of life, we exist as a bubble made of a single layer of cells with no openings, called a blastula. But soon after that, a stage called gastrulation occurs where one side of our cell bubble starts to sink into itself (called invagination) until it forms a sort of cup or bowl shape that is now two layers thick. The original outer layer of cells will eventually become skin and the nervous system (ectoderm), and the inner layer of cells will become the digestive system (endoderm). Cells that develop between the ectoderm and endoderm are called the mesoderm, and they become our innards. The opening of the gastrula "cup" is what becomes the anus, and later in development a separate opening is created that becomes the mouth.

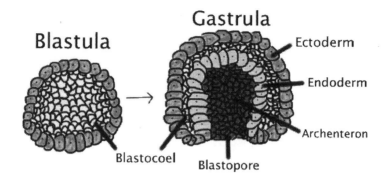

What is interesting here is that the space that is created for the digestive system is a continuation of the outer part of the embryo, which will become the skin. Even in fully formed humans, though we have valves and sphincters to control the flow of food and fluid through the digestive system, nothing that goes in the mouth ever really goes inside the body. It is only through absorption of substances filtered through the intestinal lining that something enters the body's inner parts. Thus it is simply a compartmentalization of the ecosystem rather than a distinctly different ecosystem. What many consider the inside of the body is technically *still* the outside if it is in the gut. If this still is unclear, consider the Lincoln tunnel that connects New York City to New Jersey. It is built 30 meters below the water of the Hudson River. However, while a car is driving through the tunnel, would you consider it to be inside the Hudson River or outside of the Hudson River? Although the tunnel allows the car to travel through the river, it never is inside the river. Humans, like the Hudson, have a tunnel that runs through us called the alimentary canal – otherwise referred to as the GI tract or gut. The microbes of the gut are on the outside of its lining, so they are technically outside the body. They act through signaling pathways to effect absorption of substances and signaling to the body and brain in ways that can affect everything from inflammation to cancer.

All that is to say that the human body, like a house, may have an indoors and outdoors. However, what is considered indoors isn't actually "inside" the house. The beams (like bones) are inside the house, the insulation (like fat) is inside the house, and the plumbing (like the cardiovascular system) is inside the house. The inhabitants, however, they are not inside the house…they are in the gut.

THE "INSIDE" TRUTH OF THE GBS AXIS

Although this book focuses on the skin biome, we have learned through our study of embryology that it is critical to respect and take advantage of the inherent interconnection among the skin biome, the gut biome, and the brain as both a unified set and individual elements. Only in this way can we optimize their connection and keep our skin healthy and youthful as we age. As we saw in Chapter 2, this gut-brain-skin (GBS) axis is mostly discussed regarding how the gut biome and the brain are interconnected. The humanoid component of the gut is, of course, controlled by the brain in many aspects since our brain stem acts to regulate the digestive system. There are also other ways the brain affects the gut such as through the medulla oblongata when our body needs to vomit. Likewise, there is a signal from our digestive tract to our brain when we are feeling full or bloated. But what is of more interest to the topic of the biome is the way the non-humanoid components of the gut biome can cause changes to the way we think and act, which happens mainly through the metabolism of the substances we ingest such as food, drugs, and whatever else we partake of.

We often forget that when we eat or drink, it not only affects our human cells but can affect our microbiomes as well. And just as different types of nutrients affect our human cells, the same is true of the micro-biome. It is important to know that the environment you provide the gut affects what grows there, and the food sources you give those microbes can have a huge impact, not only on their health and survival but also on yours due to the significant impact that by-products created by the microbes can have on your body after they eat the foods you do.

A prime example of this is ingestion of dairy products that are rich in the sugar called lactose. Adult animals are not meant to ingest their mother's milk after they're weaned, so the gene for lactase, which is the enzyme for the digestion of lactose, is typically turned off so we don't waste the body's energy making something it doesn't need. However, some of the microbes in our digestive tract can digest lactose, and with large amounts of lactose being digested into fatty acids and gasses such as methane and carbon dioxide, bowel irritation occurs, and the outcome is often painful and unpleasant, as any lactose-intolerant person will tell you.

One way to think about how what you eat affects your brain via your gut microbiome is by looking at the process of fermentation of grapes, by yeast, to make wine. It isn't just any molecule in the grapes or the yeast itself that makes you drunk from wine; it is the by-product of the yeast eating the sugars and converting them into alcohol that does that. In your gut, your microbes are constantly taking the food you eat and creating new molecules you never ingested but can have major implications on your health, for better or for worse.

The same can be said for the drugs we take. It wasn't until recently that we began to pay attention to the way our microbiomes metabolize potential oral drugs. We learned that drug potency can be affected by the types and numbers of microbes in the gut as well as the other foods we eat, which in turn create other molecules that can interact with those drugs. This is a two-edged sword. Our gut microbes can cause the acceleration of neurological diseases such as Parkinson's, depending on our diet and the microbiome metabolites created in the gut. But it can also affect drugs for diseases such as Parkinson's, making drugs either more or less potent. We are beginning to see more and more microbiome testing when deciding how to treat certain disease states. Unfortunately, it is not happening fast enough to help many people who are currently suffering from these conditions. But given the trajectory, it may soon be more common. And we must consider the same phenomenon for how the skin biome is affected by what we place onto to it and what implications that has on the GBS axis.

THE "OUTSIDE" TRUTH OF THE GBS AXIS

Just like the gut, the skin has a direct connection to the nervous system. That makes sense since they both come from the same ectodermic cells in early embryological development. Here are some examples of that:

- When you experience a strong emotional feeling such as extreme joy, fear, or sexual arousal, your sympathetic nervous system tells the tiny arrector pili muscles that surround each hair follicle unit to contract and raise the hairs. The result is goose bumps (fun fact: one of the technical names for goose bumps is a piloerection, so next time you get goose bumps, tell your friends you are having a piloerection and see what their response is).

- When you get embarrassed, you blush and feel heat on your face due to the sympathetic nervous system telling the blood vessels in your skin to dilate, bringing more warm, red blood closer to the surface of your skin.

- When you are nervous, you might find that your feet, palms, and underarms sweat profusely. Again, it's the nervous system telling the sweat glands of your skin to do that.

The list goes on. Just like with the gut, it makes sense that this communication isn't a one-way street as our skin sends signals to the brain that can cause all sorts of physiological changes. If skin gets hot then we sweat, and if it gets cold then we shiver. So, it stands to reason that the balance of the skin biome can have implications to the GBS axis just like the gut As we have discussed in great detail, the skin biome is vast in size and complex, so let's explore what is similar and what is different about the skin and gut biomes and how that may affect their interaction with the nervous system as well as with each other.

THERE'S NO PLACE LIKE BIOME

Both gut and skin biomes are comprised of these three main components: (1) human epithelium cells that interface with the external environment (whether it is the cavity of the digestive system or the outside world), (2) the microbiota, and (3) the environment that is unique to each biome and acts to shape and is shaped by the human and microbial members of the biome. To again use the analogy of a house, our skin biome would be the outside walls of the home and the environment around them, and the gut biome would be the inside walls and the environment around them. We could take the analogy to a quite literal place and say that the microbes that grow on the outside walls of your house are very likely different than what grows on the interior walls of your house. That's because (1) the materials used to make both sets of walls are slightly different or sealed differently, and (2) the environment is likely quite different in the two spaces (unless you are like our friend Jackson and leave your home exposed to nature).

However, there are also similarities between those walls. They both must provide some degree of structure. They both need to be somewhat pliable so they can withstand the expansion and contraction of seasonal temperature changes in order not to crack. Most importantly, they both provide access to the inner workings of your home with conduits such as light switches, electrical outlets, faucets, and the like. You might notice, however, that you have far more of these conduits on the inside of your home than on the outside, and the conduits on the outside tend to have more robust fittings or materials around them to prevent degradation upon exposure to elements that the indoor fixtures are not typically exposed to.

This is a great way to think about the similarities and differences of the skin and gut biomes. Let's explore this further by also comparing each element of those biomes to the home:

The Human "Walls" of the Biomes

- *Similarities:* The walls of your digestive system and your skin are both made to do at least two main things: (1) keep bad things out and (2) keep and bring good things in. Both start with a type of cell called an epithelial cell. In your skin, it is the epidermis; in your gut, the epithelial cells are mostly absorptive cells (entero-cytes) with scattered goblet cells and occasional enteroendocrine cells. Deeper in the walls are more structural layers of tissue that are more fibrous and dense, such as the dermis of the skin and the submuscosa of the digestive tract. Both biomes have "wall" structures that are designed to separate the exterior from the interior of the body.

- *Differences:* Like a house, the walls of the biomes are comprised of *similar* materials, but they are not the *same*. They are differentiated based on the overall requirements of the particular wall or barrier. One of the most important things to do on the outside walls of our home is waterproof them. That is where the analogy is a little off since we do this to our homes to prevent water from entering and damaging the structure. In our skin, the opposite is true; we want to keep water from *leaving* the body's tissues. One of the biggest differences between the walls of the skin and gut biomes is the development of the stratum corneum, or the thin outermost layer of the skin. This layer is comprised of flattened, epidermal cells that have basically been mummified. That makes them tough and leathery so they can be used along with sebaceous secretions as a sort of brick-and-mortar barrier. This structure also helps reflect and absorb UV rays from the sun.[2] [3] This part is important since it is far better to damage the stratum corneum with solar radiation since it eventually just falls off the body than to expose your delicate epidermal cells. This is another reason you should *not* be exfoliating too much.

The walls of the gut, on the other hand, are more specialized in absorbing nutrients from the food we take in and bringing those nutrients into the body. The skin does that as well but in a much less capacity.

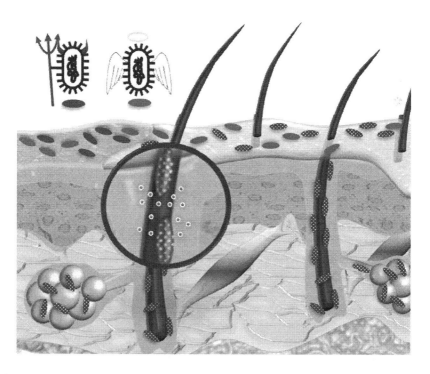

The Human "Fixtures" of the Biomes

- *Similarities:* Just like we have light switches and electrical outlets both inside and outside our homes, there is a similar concept within the biomes of the gut and skin. That is the nervous system. The skin and the gut both have nerve endings that interact with the central nervous system.

- *Differences:* Both the skin and the gut have "fixtures" that could be compared to faucets of sorts. However, although we have these types of structures in both biomes, they have somewhat different makeups. It's worth noting that part of what coats both biomes' walls is similar in concept but different in composition. In the skin we have sebum and sweat that is secreted by the sebaceous and sweat glands; in the gut we have mucus that is secreted by goblet cells. Both serve to keep the biomes lubricated and moving in the right direction. There are other differences as well that we won't get into on the "fixture" front. Needless to say, most of those differences go along with the overall main difference in functions between the biomes.

The Microbiomes of the Biomes

- We won't get too much into the differences between the micro-biomes of the skin and gut. But what we do want to convey is that there are a couple of interesting similarities between how the microbiomes of each biome function and interact with the human cells. Those similarities are the production of biofilms by the microbes and how that plays into whether a microbe becomes a permanent resident (engrafts) or remains a visitor (planktonic).

Biofilms are gel-like substances that microbes secrete under certain circumstances in order to claim their territory. Basically, it is a way a colony of microbes build their own little home inside their human homes (I guess that makes humans more of a city— really stretching the analogy here). In this way, microbes tend to engraft onto the skin. Microbes that cannot establish on the skin are considered planktonic (or transient) and thus are not likely to have time to make a biofilm. However, there is some research emerging that suggests that some microbes can hijack the biofilm homes of established symbiotic microbes, which may be how some microbiome-related issues arise. It seems that some visitors just don't know when it is time to leave.

Biofilms are often referred to medically as a nuisance since they can make it hard to get rid of unwanted microbes that are causing an illness. That is like how *Staphlococcus aureus* can claim certain areas of skin in those with atopic dermatitis. And just like we do with our homes, microbes try to make *their* biofilm homes as cozy as possible for themselves, secreting certain substances they like, some that also affects us. They even have a type of security system they set up by secreting molecules into the biofilm that keep other specific microbes away while allowing others in. A great example of this is how *C. acnes* strains can secrete one of a few types of molecules into their biofilms inside the hair follicles. *C. acnes* also secrete a huge amount of antioxidants into their biofilms since it makes it more comfortable for them to live. So, it's a win-win in that skin biome example that is if it is the correct strain of *C. acnes*, of course.

THE BIOME'S IMMUNITY CONNECTION

We have discussed that the skin and the gut biome are connected to the brain, and the health of both biomes can impact your overall health by how they impact their local ecosystems and how they affect the central nervous system that impacts nearly the whole body. Another facet of the connectivity among the skin, gut, and brain is through the immune system. As we discussed in Chapter 2, the skin is the largest immune organ of the body with tens of millions of immune cells living throughout the skin, especially surrounding the hair follicles that don't have the stratum corneum barrier as protection. That makes sense because the skin is exposed at every moment to billions of new microbes as we interact with our environment. As already mentioned, bacteria in the skin biome can affect the activity of the skin's immune cells quite extensively. That can manifest in the ways immune cells monitor the skin, what microbes they accept or reject, whether they create inflammation in the skin, and consequently how your skin looks and feels.

We also know that the gut has a very robust immune presence. That also makes perfect sense since the lining of the gut (the gut walls) is exposed to a large amount of microbial contact each time we ingest food and fluids. So based on what is going on in the gut biome, we can experience health or malaise, depending on what we ingest and how that affects both our human cells and the associated microbial metabolism. Like the skin, different kinds of microbes or food sources can cause the immune cells in the gut to manifest in either quiescence or inflammation, and that in turn manifests in either health or disease.

These facts are important because the immune system isn't static. For example, inflammation in one part of the body is not necessarily contained to that particular area. There have been hundreds of studies that have examined how inflammatory skin issues such as acne vulgaris, psoriasis, rosacea, alopecia areata, and hidradenitis suppurativa are highly associated with dysbiosis of gut microbiome.[4,5,6] Most of the research has focused on how inflammation caused by the gut biome may contribute to systemic inflammation and therefore inflammatory skin issues. One example is a study that correlated the eradication of a species of pathogenic bacteria called *H. pylori* and how ridding the gut of such bacteria reduces the symptoms of *both* rosacea and the known gut issues associated with that species.[7] Unfortunately, less thought has been given to the reciprocal association with systemic inflammation. In essence, if gut dysbiosis can cause skin issues, can skin dysbiosis cause gut issues?

Most people would concede that diet can play a large role in skin health, given the interactions of the skin and gut biomes.[8] Low-fiber intake in Western societies is thought to be one of the major causes of depletion of the human gastrointestinal microbiota and subsequent increases in chronic systemic diseases such as obesity, cardiovascular disease, type II diabetes, and colon cancer.[9] Diets high in meats are also thought to contribute to systemic diseases from the effects on the microbes in the gut biome. Much of that is due to the loss of short chain fatty acids that are created when the gut microbes eat dietary fibers that our human cells cannot digest or absorb. Just like in the skin, short chain fatty acids such as butyric acid and propionic acid are extremely important to systemic health. Additionally, research on a diet's association with acne has shown that certain trends in dietary habits show a strong association with the intensity of the disease. For instance, diets low in glycemic index (i.e., less processed sugars, grains, and starches) and high in omega-3 fatty acid supplements or γ-linoleic acid supplements have shown significant reductions in the amounts and intensity of acne lesions.[10]

Dr. Day: Many of my patients who come in with flares of skin conditions, especially psoriasis, find that a specific set of changes in their diet can impact their skin and often their joints as well. We know that about 30% of people with psoriasis also have psoriatic arthritis. There seems to be a gut-skin connection and a gut-joint connection that causes this. Bacterial cell wall products and bacterial by-products can leak into the body and trigger inflammation, which leads to the signs and symptoms of psoriasis and psoriatic arthritis in those who have a genetic predisposition to the disease. By eliminating alcohol and hot peppers (anything spicy hot on the tongue) and adding supplements such as duozyme and quercetin, many of these patients have been able to have long-term remission and clear skin.

BI-HOME IMPROVEMENT

All in all, the gut and the skin are very connected. They are guardians of your body and act as gatekeepers to anything that may attempt to enter from the outside world. The ways they fulfill these duties are quite similar, even with their very different overall functions for the body. It is the immune system that connects them in the most direct manner. If we stop to think about all we've learned about the ecosystems that comprise the biomes of the skin and the gut, it stands to reason that the culprit for disruptions or dysbiosis in either biome is likely due to the addition of either food sources or foreign microbes rather than residents of the biome. And if the residents do cause problems, it is often because we have changed something about the environment that contributes to a change in their behavior. We can again liken this to our analogy of our body as a house. If we leave food out, a visitor (e.g., fruit flies, cockroaches) may end up as a residential nuisance. If we don't leave food out, they either never come (at least in appreciable amounts) or simply go away.

Our analogy is just that—an analogy—and the human body is much more complex than any house structure or components. It is a good comparison, however, because it shows how the biomes can function harmoniously if there is proper bi-home (get it, biome) maintenance or if home improvements are made. While hygiene and what you put on the skin is important for the skin biome, diet is also very important for the reasons we have described. Many "gurus" may attribute certain fad diets (e.g., raw, vegetarian, vegan) to better skin, but none of these diets have been clinically shown to be uniquely beneficial. That being said, we do know that balanced diets that contain essential nutrients; are low in (preferably devoid of) processed foods, are low in dairy, high in low glycemic index foods, and high in foods rich in omega-3 and omega-6 fatty acids have been shown to have great benefits for your skin and overall systemic health. The GBS axis, it's all connected folks.

Interestingly, there is evidence that will bring this chapter to an ironic conclusion. Crickets (a bug, of all things) meet most of the requirements of a skin-healthy food since they are rich in protein, polyunsaturated fats such as omega-3s, vitamins, minerals, and fiber, and may help promote gut health. And they are more environmentally friendly than meat farming, to boot. I guess we owe Jackson an apology.

CHAPTER 9

THE HOLOBIONT PHILOSOPHY

No matter how clean you think you are,
you have billions of bacteria on your skin.
How they affect your life depends on how you affect theirs.
—Thomas Hitchcock

Let's begin this final chapter by reimagining that lush, life-filled land-scape we conjured up when we started this journey together. Try to let your mind recreate the sights, the sounds, even the smells of this imaginary ecosystem we created. Recall looking at the vast fields of tall grass with the occasional smattering of colorful wildflowers and the green, leafy forest in the distance. Recall the sounds of the wind as it rushed through the trees and onto the field, and the orchestra of birds and insects as they went about their daily business. Think of the smell of the fresh outdoor air, unpolluted and sweetened with the fragrances of the flowers and grass.

Now consider that you have been left solely in charge of caring for that ecosystem. How do you go about doing so? If you have been paying attention to the philosophy of this book, you likely would answer, "I would just leave it alone and let it exist in balance." And that would be exactly the best thing for any natural ecosystem. However, when it comes to our skin, we don't live in a world where we can leave our skin biome in its natural state. We have to deal with factors that humans add to the environment, especially in urban living situations. We are exposed to pollution, many of us wear makeup, and we put on antiperspirant. We go to the gym and shower frequently with soap. We wear clothes and quickly go from one temperature extreme to another as we go from indoors to outside and back. So in order for our analogy to work for this particular chapter, we must change our scenario a bit.

Reimagine that the landscape created in your mind is actually in the middle of a major metropolitan city. Now you don't have the luxury of just letting it exist. You have to deal with a more complicated scenario where there are visitors that come and go frequently. The foliage is pruned and trimmed to make it appealing to the visitors and to meet city requirements. You have to clean up any garbage those visitors leave behind and provide places they can sit and visit. You will need barriers that block the places these visitors shouldn't go so they don't disturb the ecosystem. To make matters worse, you have to deal with pollution from cars that surround the park and how the water supply is fluoridated. How might that visitor traffic, air pollution, and fluoridated water affect our landscape?

Now imagine that in order to care for this landscape, you are only allowed to feed and trim the foliage but are expressly forbidden from caring for the creatures that live there. You are also told that you must use pesticides to keep the flies away from tourists, and that the only source of nutrients you can use must also contain those pesticides that are just fine for the plants but poisonous to the wildlife. So, you attempt to care for this city area in this manner, but in doing so, you kill the bees that pollinate the foliage and eradicate the earthworms that aerate and fortify the soil. As a result, you lose the birds that feed on the insects and worms, and their songs disappear from the landscape. While you are able to maintain the foliage somewhat through chemicals and fertilizers, lack of pollination allows them to yield little to no fruits, so the squirrels and other small animals migrate elsewhere. You are left with an incomplete ecosystem that has the land and the foliage but none of the creatures that make it thrive.

This is the metaphorical equivalent of those "germ-free" animals that were created in the 1940s—the animals that could survive but not thrive.

The visitors that simply pass through might see green trees and grass and maybe some flowers that had to be constantly replanted because none of the natural ones would bloom. What they don't see is that it is a version of an ecosystem, incomplete and held in place through artificial means. The real question is whether it matters to them that the ecosystem in the park is not thriving as long as it is nice enough for a mid-day stroll.

THE HOLOBIONT RATIONALE

The above fantasy was designed to allude to the way the modern way of life has affected our bodies' biomes, especially the skin and gut biomes. We have adopted a modern way of life that has allowed us a significantly extended lifespan compared to our ancestors—at least those documented historically. Modern sanitation allows us to live free of the fear of things we take for granted but that may have killed us in years past. They include clean drinking water free of pathogens, as well as preserved foods through refrigeration and preservatives that are free of potentially harmful toxins and microbes such as salmonella. We have antibiotics so very few people will die from a simple cut or scrape that may have been a death sentence in years gone by. We have topical inventions such as sunscreens to protect us from the excess radiation of the sun.

All these things are good, but like everything in life, they are good only under the right circumstances, and overuse can be problematic. Things like fluoride, food preservatives, and antibiotics have allowed us to raise the standard of living in the world; however, we must look at the overall implications to see the impact they can have on human ecology over the long term. Toxicologists have looked at these substances to see if they are harmful in certain concentrations and deemed safe up to certain levels for either consumption or topical application. However, if you recall from our earlier discussion, there are many things that scientists and physicians had initially deemed safe and effective but later found to not be so. We do not believe the use of fluoridated water, food preservatives, or antibiotics is a bad thing, nor do we believe they should not be used. However, we do believe that we should be wise in the way we use them and that every so often we take new science that is emerging and check our paradigms against what we are learning.

This is the case with the Holobiont Philosophy. Until recently, toxicologists would assess whether certain chemicals were toxic to human cells. But that doesn't necessarily take into account how those substances may indirectly affect human cells via their microflora. For instance, fluoridated water has been thought to help reduce tooth decay in children and adults and has been deemed safe for human consumption in toxicology reports. However, how does fluoride do this? Fluoride is thought to act through a couple of methods—by strengthening enamel and by its strong antimicrobial activity. It is the latter that is relevant to our discussion since it begs the question of what constant imbibing of fluoridated water does to the body's biomes. And does it really prevent tooth decay? A meta-analysis of 155 studies on whether fluoridated water truly prevents tooth decay found that there is really not much, if any, evidence that it does.[1]

Additionally, too much fluoride has been linked to neurological disease in developing children.[2] That is not to say that we should not implement the use of fluoride in our oral hygiene, but perhaps we should rethink how much of it we are exposed to, in what ways we are exposed to it, and what the level of exposure may have on the rest of our body's biomes due to the antimicrobial activity of fluoride. Do the potential benefits of adding fluoride to drinking water outweigh the potential for harm? Since we have not really seen the true benefits of providing people with fluoride in their water, we then must ask whether one day we will realize the true potential harms and whether the current practices may change from the status quo and join the outdated practices of yesteryear, like bloodletting, as niche treatment rather than one of broad implementation.

Another thought to mull over is our food preservation methods. I don't think anyone would argue against the fact that fresh food is better for us. However, most people do not have time to shop frequently enough at a farmers' market to always keep the pantry stocked with the freshest foods. We have food preservatives that allow us to stock foods at room temperature and under refrigeration for relatively long periods of time. And while this is convenient, we need to think about what the implications of those preservatives are on our overall health. Sure, I'd rather have preserved food than spoiled food with salmonella in it, but the best option would be to have fresh food or at least a preservation method that employs something I know will not harm my biome.

Most preservatives are meant to be antimicrobial, so we have to wonder how that affects our overall biomes of the gut and therefore ultimately our bodies. On top of that, crops are being genetically modified to be resistant to microbes, but we're finding that in many cases, it also affects the nutritional value and quality of the food. We know that Western diets are largely associated with conditions such as obesity and diabetes. And while that is in part due to the macronutrient makeup of the Western diet (high in refined foods and saturated fats), it is also the inclusion of preservatives and other ingredients such as emulsifiers and artificial sweeteners that allow us to make more complicated foods in less time and with less effort. These food additives have been linked to digestive diseases such as colitis and overall gut dysbiosis-associated inflammatory issues. [3,4,5]

So should we stop using preservatives? No, but some preservatives seem to have less potential for biome harm than others. The issue is that those preservatives are not always the most inexpensive or convenient for manufacturers of food products to use.

Now let's talk about antibiotics, a very two-edged sword. Antibiotics are a miracle sent to humanity. The fact that microbes create substances that keep other pathogenic microbes in check is something we should explore and exploit as we have these last several decades. However, we have become irresponsible in how we have wielded this microbial weapon. Rather than look for other remedies first, society has been guilty of throwing antibiotics at too many issues, and some of them have nothing to do with bacteria. As mentioned in other chapters, antibiotics play a huge role in medicine but are often overused and can lead not only to dysbiosis of the skin and gut microbiome but also to the emergence of resistant strains, potentially making them less effective when they are most needed. There are strong efforts in place to use antibiotics in a more strategic and selective way based on what we now know.

All these examples have much in common. They all show how we have some wonderful technologies in science and medicine that have allowed us to bring humanity two steps forward, but somewhere we have crossed a line where something—be it convenience, greed, ignorance, or ineptitude—has taken us a step backward. The whole rationale behind the Holobiont Philosophy is not necessarily to remove all these modern marvels from our daily routines (although some things may need to be removed) but simply to make sure the things we do use are being utilized with educated intention, applying what we do know in order to affect our holobiont in the best way possible.

FINDING THE BALANCE IN YOUR BIOME

With all we know, we can now consider what ways we can apply the Holobiont Philosophy to our daily lives in order to give us the very best biomes possible in the modern world. For the skin biome, which is the major emphasis of this book, we must make sure that all skin care products and treatments fall under the biome-care umbrella, as discussed in Chapter 7. However, since the skin, brain, and gut biomes are connected to each other and through the immune system to the entire body, that leads us to one seminal truth—to truly care for the skin, you must care for the holobiont, which is the entire body, the entire microbiome, and the environments that house them all. That is not an insignificant task and requires you to take a look at all your daily habits to see if they fall under this philosophy. We don't claim to lead immaculate lives that meticulously follow this philosophy, but we do aspire to such. It is a daily challenge to evaluate all you do and bring it into a balance of what you can do and what you should do, and then make it what you want to do.

Outside-In Hygiene

We won't spend too much time on what your biome-care regimen should look like since that is outlined pretty well in Chapters 7 and 8. However, we do want to rehash some of the basic principles and expand on a couple of them.

Sun protection: We really need to dig into sun protection a bit more since there are some principles that most people simply do not know about. The UV rays the sun produces are necessary for some of our body's functions. But like most things in life, excess UV radiation is quite bad for the skin biome. One good thing about the sun's rays is that they turn the porphyrins that pathogenic *C. acnes* acne strains produce into free radicals and can help kill some of those bad strains. The bad news is that unless you have *C. acnes defendens* strains to fill the void, it is likely that the troublesome strains will return.

Free radicals are damaging to our biomes in general, so we don't want to repeat this pattern too often. Regarding the rest of the skin biome, it is crucial to protect your skin from excess UV rays from the sun and other human-made sources, no matter how glorious the sun feels on your skin when you're outside sitting on a beach. Not only do UVB rays cause burns, but UVA rays can penetrate deeply into the skin and cause damage to your collagen and cellular DNA through free radicals. The result is premature aging and damaged skin. But your skin does have ways to protect itself—natural sunscreens, if you will.

As we've already discussed, the stratum corneum is the outermost layer of skin. There are many companies that proclaim that it's just a dead outer layer and serves no purpose, and they make products whose sole purpose is to help get rid of that layer through exfoliation. What most people don't know is that the stratum corneum is a haven for most of the surface microbes of the skin and helps prevent excess water loss from the skin. But it also plays a big part in our defense against the sun.[6] While you might consider that outer portion of the stratum corneum to be expendable, what you might not know is that UV radiation is partially absorbed by some of the molecules in that layer. It has also been postulated that once that layer of the stratum corneum is removed, the integrity of the layer is compromised and now less effective in protecting the skin. It is important that we always have an outer expendable layer that can absorb damage, with a fresh layer underneath that can emerge as the damaged layers slough off. If we leave little to no stratum corneum, then the next in line for UV damage is the actual epidermal cells. Additionally, the stratum corneum isn't as thick as you might believe, especially on your face. While it can be quite thick on your soles and palms (0.5–1 mm), it is only about 0.05–0.1 mm thick on the face. That is about as thick as the sheet of paper this book may be printed on.

Dr. Day: Janice (not her real name) came in complaining of irritated and overly sensitive skin. She said any product she applied instantly burned her skin, and she had a bag full of products to show me proof of her attempts to heal her skin. We went through each one, and not surprisingly, common ingredients in many of her products were either physical or chemical exfoliants. She was wearing away her stratum corneum, exposing the under-lying layers and allowing any product she applied to penetrate more quickly than designed, often leading to burning, stinging, and redness. Her skin was dry, broken out, and very red. We reorganized her skin care routine to a more biome-friendly one, and within a week, she was on the road to clear, beautiful, healthy skin.

Part of what makes the stratum corneum so protective from the sun is the copious amounts of antioxidants put there by both you (your sebaceous glands) and your microbiome (*C. acnes*). One of the ways UV affects the skin adversely is by the creation of free radicals around and within skin cells. Once these free radicals are created, it is imperative that they be quickly dealt with by antioxidants that are specifically made to deal with them. Otherwise, those free radicals will find other molecules to mess with instead, molecules whose functions are more essential to cell function and integrity. These include molecules such as structural proteins, enzymes, and, most importantly, DNA. That is how UV radiation contributes to photoaging and cancers of the skin.

The oils of the skin are filled with antioxidants from your own sebaceous glands as well as those such as RoxP from your resident *C. acnes*. That is why the way you cleanse and exfoliate is of the utmost importance for general skin health but also for protection from the environment, including UV radiation from the sun. Melanin produced by our melanocytes is also of prime importance, but for those of us who are naturally fair-skinned, melanin tends to be produced mostly as a reaction to UV damage. That means if you get a tan, it's because your skin has been damaged and your body is pulling out all the stops to avoid further damage. The goal should be to preserve your first line of defense—your stratum corneum and all the antioxidants it contains.

Next, you should consider wearing sunscreen as another layer of defense against solar radiation. This topic can get a bit controversial. There is an array of chemicals that can be placed on the skin in order to absorb and reflect UV rays away from the structures of your biome. They are basically two kinds—organic sunscreens and inorganic sunscreens. These are chemical terms and may not be what you think. Inorganic sunscreens are typically known as mineral sunscreens and are usually either zinc oxide or titanium dioxide. Some refer to organic sunscreens as chemical sunscreens. They are more abundant as far as the number of options to choose from, and they are often preferred from a cosmetic standpoint since they blend into the skin well and tend to be invisible. However, they are becoming quite controversial with regard to human health as well as the health of the environment.

There are some controversial studies that claim organic sunscreens are partially responsible for bleaching (death) of coral reefs in highly popular tourist areas. While this is currently highly debatable since the publication with those claims has been called into question regarding its credibility, organic sunscreens have also been found by an FDA study to leach into human plasma. Whether that has any bearing on the health of our biomes, skin, or anything else is yet to be determined. For now, the FDA is asking sunscreen manufacturers for more information, but it is not reversing its approval of those sunscreen ingredients.

However, many people opt to use inorganic sunscreens such as zinc oxide primarily to avoid these issues mentioned above. But they also have their issues. Though most of the mechanisms by which inorganic sunscreens protect the skin are through absorption of UV radiation,[7,8] they tend to reflect the visible spectrum of light. That results in a white cast to the skin, making those who apply the sunscreens appear paler in tone (or bluish in tone for those with more pigmented skin). That is, of course, a cosmetic issue and does not affect the effectiveness of the sunscreen. However, if someone does not like how they look when they're wearing sunscreen, they are less likely to use it regularly. As such, one must decide which of these issues if of most importance to them.

While these sunscreens may be effective at protecting human cells from radiation, we must also consider the effect the formulation has on the microbiome of the skin. Remember, some of these sunscreen ingredients (e.g., zinc oxide) can be very antimicrobial. By applying any significantly potent antimicrobial, you run the risk of potential dysbiosis with chronic application. You would thus be trading one issue for another. However, the good news is that most sunscreens with inorganic active ingredients use film-forming agents to ensure that the layer of the sun-protective elements are even and dispersed properly. They tend to stay on the skin's outermost surface, and while they may affect the more planktonic (free-floating) microbes on the outermost stratum corneum, they should not affect the engrafted portions of the skin microbiome very much—another reason the biofilms secreted by our skin's commensal and symbiotic microbes are useful for biome health, as they too help protect engrafted microbes from topical antimicrobials.

However, that doesn't mean all formulations with inorganic sunscreen actives will not affect the microbiomes of the skin. Formulations contain much more than just the actives that are bound by the film formers. If you are concerned about the antimicrobial properties of a mineral sunscreen, you should find a formulation that contains a coated zinc or titanium since that can make it less antimicrobial (depending on the coating) and more compatible with the biome. Additionally, you can look for a biomecare-centric moisturizer that provides a barrier between the biome and the sunscreen applied last. That way you can protect the biome in the most comprehensive way without knowing whether any particular sunscreen is biome-compatible.

And then there are those who shun the use of sunscreens, claiming they limit the body's natural production of vitamin D that occurs when the skin is exposed to UVB rays from the sun. While it is true that sunlight exposure to the skin is important to the body for multiple reasons (e.g., production of vitamin D), that should definitely not preclude anyone from not protecting their skin on a regular basis from UV radiation. There have been several experimental studies in labs using artificial UV radiation to observe the effects of sunscreen on vitamin D production, and those experiments did show that sunscreen applied in proper amounts can actually mitigate the production of vitamin D in the skin. Dozens of observational studies have shown that daily applications of moderate SPF (sun protection factor) less than 30 do not affect the body's production of vitamin D in any significant way. Some self-reported studies actually claimed more vitamin D production.[9] It should be noted that these field study results are likely due to a few reasons: (1) people tend to not wear sunscreen correctly, so the full SPF of the product is typically not achieved; (2) those who wear sunscreen may spend more time in the sun, allowing for more exposure to UV radiation and thus more potential for vitamin D production; and (3) the studies only looked at the use of moderate SPF (less than 30).

Something that should be mentioned in the context of these studies is that they did not evaluate the ever-rising SFP numbers that companies are producing. At the time of this writing, it is quite typical for companies to produce and promote SFP 50 in their sunscreen products. Much of that is due to marketing pressure, but it is also because people are spending long periods of time in the sun and not properly applying sunscreen. It is thought that a higher SPF will give greater protection and allow for safer outdoor activities. While it may be that proper use of high SPF sunscreen could inhibit the body's ability to create vitamin D when the sunscreen is used properly, we still advise using sunscreen during outdoor activities that last longer than 15 minutes, especially in mid-day. That is because unless you are *properly* wearing a high SPF every minute, it is likely that you are receiving enough incidental sunlight on a daily basis to cover your vitamin D needs. And when you weigh the risks of skin damage and the premature aging that goes with it (think leathery, blotchy skin), as well as skin cancer from the sun and making up for any lost vitamin D, it really is a no-brainer to opt to protect the skin. After all, when it comes to vitamin D, there are supplements that can help make up the difference. That leads us to our next topic.

Inside Out – Medications, Supplementation, and Diet

The strong connection between the microbiomes of the gut and the skin leads us to reinforce the importance of what you ingest and how that can affect the skin biome. That doesn't just mean your diet; it also means the medications and the supplements you take.

Medications: Keep in mind that just like our human cells can metabolize molecules, so can the microbes of the skin and gut. That means a molecule that can have great medicinal value to human cells may or may not be affected by the microbes, depending on (1) what microbes are in your biomes and (2) if the microbes can metabolize any particular medication. Since certain substances that microbes produce can affect what substances our human cells produce, it has been observed that our microbes can even affect the way we metabolize certain drugs. There are dozens of drugs that have become less effective or even more toxic in the presence of the wrong gut microbes. They include common drugs such as acetaminophen for pain, L-dopa for Parkinson's disease, and statins for high cholesterol.

So what can you do about that? How would you know if the medication you are taking is being influenced by the wrong microbes in the gut? Currently, that is very hard to know since most physicians are still not looking at this problem. However, as mentioned before, testing the microbes of the various biomes of the body is catching on as more and more clinicians are becoming aware of the interconnectedness of humans and microbiomes. For now, what you can do is foster a symbiotic biome in the gut by adopting the Holobiont Philosophy for all biomes, skin, and gut. If you need help with this, it is best to talk to your physician, and if your doctor doesn't know, perhaps they can help you find a doctor who does.

Supplementation: Are there truly any supplements that can benefit the skin biome? Despite much marketing hype, we know that most things that are digested do not target the skin biome specifically but are metabolized and used throughout the entire body. They include supplements that are popularly sold as skin-centric such as hydrolyzed collagen. Unlike the claims you might read in the marketing of these supplements, there is a dearth of evidence that any particular type of protein supplement, including collagen protein, is digested into peptides and amino acids that are added to the same pool of nutrients for all body parts. It's not going to be directed at only your skin— there is no evidence that your body can direct amino acids from specific protein sources to move on up to a specific body part any more than doing cardio can reduce fat in a specific preferential area.

However, there is some emerging evidence that suggests an overall benefit to connective tissue (including skin) when taking oral supplements high in proteins and certain amino acids such as hydrolyzed collagen peptides. We know that some foods high in collagen such as bone broth, fish, chicken, egg whites, leafy greens, and the algae spirulina are associated with a healthy diet.

But, not all forms of collagen are readily bioavailable when ingested, adding controversy to the value of oral supplemental collagen. Because native collagen is such a large and complex protein, the molecule in its entirety cannot pass directly from the digestive tract to the bloodstream. Instead, collagen must first be denatured by heat (turned into gelatin), and then hydrolyzed (cut by enzymes) into short fragments only two or three amino acids long. Fifty percent of these di-and tripeptides are composed of the amino acids proline, glycine, and hydroxyproline, the amino acids that give collagen its unique structure. In this form, the collagen fragments are water soluble and easily absorbed and distributed in the human body—studies have traced these fragments after ingestion and have confirmed that they appear in the bloodstream and then integrate into the skin.[10]

There is no reason that these amino acids need to come from collagen, but as with all protein supplementation it does provide the cells of the body more resources to make proteins. However, it has been proposed that collagen peptides have additional utility in their di- and tri-peptide forms as they have been observed to bind to fibroblast membrane receptors and trigger signaling cascades for new collagen synthesis in cell culture. In addition, hydrolyzed collagen peptides have different functional properties, such as antioxidant and antimicrobial activity, depending on the degree of hydrolysis and the enzyme used. Specifically, proline-hydroxyproline dipeptides have been shown to stimulate chemotaxis and cell proliferation, enhance hyaluronic acid production, and increase water content in the stratum corneum.[11] Could these peptides be found in other types of hydrolyzed protein supplements? Sure. However, since collagen is rich in those 3 specific amino acids it raises the likelihood that the combinations of peptides will have these uniquely beneficial properties.

We concede that the benefits of oral supplementation as a clinical tool still need much more investigation. Despite this, oral collagen supplements have been seen to provide some clinically demonstrated positive effects on the skin: a recent meta-analysis of 19 randomized control trials of 1,125 participants showed favorable results in skin hydration, elasticity, and wrinkles. Ingestion of hydrolyzed collagen also reduced skin aging. More controlled trials are needed, specifically on the source, form, and quality of collagen to understand the full benefits of supplemental oral collagen. So there is a potential for benefit here to oral supplementation with collagen, but as with any supplement the source and purity is important. So make sure if you do choose one, it's from a reputable company.

It should be noted that protein from certain sources such as whey protein *can indeed* affect the body differently than other proteins, although not necessarily for the better since whey protein has been associated with acne, insulin resistance, and digestive issues. That is not necessarily due to the protein but to the other molecules (e.g., lactose, etc.) that are in that particular protein mix and may adversely affect you.

Collagen supplements are just one example of supplements that claim to have skin biome benefits, but often without adequate scientific or clinical evidence. For instance, there is little evidence that supplement-ation of vitamin B3, also known as biotin, is effective for benefits to the skin or hair. However, in years past, biotin was a staple of hair and skin supplements, claiming to be essential for restoring proper skin heath. While biotin is indeed an essential vitamin for skin health, it has not been established that any significant benefits are seen by supplementing with biotin. The only groups that have been shown to receive any benefit from such supplementation are those with biotin deficiencies, which is very rare in Western diets.[12] Additionally, too much biotin in the blood can interfere with the results of some important blood tests that use biotin to attach to the molecules being tested. So not only is biotin supplementation unnecessary for healthy individuals, it also has the potential to delay the diagnosis of important health issues.

Whatever supplements you take, remember that just like drugs, they can alter the activity of both your cells and your microbiome. And just like drugs, certain supplements may be more or less effective or even toxic, depending on a person's biome ecosystem. So even though supplements can be found at any grocery store or online and you don't need a prescription to buy them, it is always best to let your personal physician know what you plan to take and let them help you determine if it is best for your situation.

The FDA and the USDA don't regulate supplements very well. There is often little to no way of knowing that the product you are ingesting is what is on the label in the amounts claimed or even if it is the same ingredient at all. It is always best to stick with highly reputable brands. That is especially important when it comes to probiotic supplements. Most of them don't survive past the acid in your stomach during normal digestion which means they have no effect in your gut and you won't get the benefits you expect. Look for encapsulated probiotics that might allow the bacteria to make it past the stomach. A balanced gut micro-biome means less systemic inflammation, which then lowers overall skin inflammation as well. Skin health is best achieved from both the outside and the inside.

Also, price alone is not the best way to know if a supplement is high quality. Some reputable brands can offer less expensive products because they sell high volumes which helps them offset the cost of goods, which they pass on to the consumer. However, the same company may sell higher-priced products because of their legitimate ingredients that are harder to find, and it costs more to make them. Other less reputable brands may try to take advantage of the higher-priced, in-demand pro-duct by providing either diluted or adulterated sources of ingredients in order to charge lower prices and benefit from impulse sales by those who fall for this trap. Always look for quality over price. With a little homework, you can figure out which brands and supplements you should explore. One resource to keep in mind is the Dietary Supplements Verification Program at USP.org.

Diet: As we discussed in the previous chapter, we know that diet can play a large role in skin health, given the interactions of the skin and gut biomes.[13] Low-fiber intake in Western societies is thought to be one of the major causes of depletion of the human gastrointestinal microbiota and subsequent increases in chronic systemic diseases such as obesity, cardiovascular disease, type II diabetes, and colon cancer.[14] Also, diets high in meats are thought to contribute to systemic diseases through the effects on the microbes in the gut biome. Much of that happens due to the loss of the short chain fatty acids that are created when the gut microbes eat dietary fibers that our human cells cannot digest or absorb. Just like the skin, short chain fatty acids such as butyric acid and propionic acid are extremely important to systemic health. Research on diet's association with acne has also shown that certain trends in dietary habits show a strong association with the intensity of the disease. For instance, diets low in their glycemic index (i.e., less processed sugars, grains, and starches) and high in omega-3 fatty acid supplements or γ-linoleic acid supplements have shown significant reductions in the amounts and intensity of acne lesions.[15] A colleague Dr Haines Ely published a fascinating article titled: "Is Psoriasis a Bowel Disease?" and made a good case that treating leaky gut could in many cases cure psoriasis. This was a big claim, but Dr. Day has had several patients follow his protocol with dramatic improvement in their condition, with many of them being able to stop their prescription treatments altogether. It doesn't work for everyone with psoriasis but there are health benefits to improving gut biome even if the psoriasis doesn't completely resolve.

Diets that are low in refined and processed foods have fewer preservatives, and are high in healthy fats, proteins, and fiber are all part of a healthy gut biome and thus a healthy skin biome as well.

Dr. Day: My dad grew up on a farm in a village outside of Tehran. He instilled in me a love of healthy foods that are as fresh as possible. He told me stories about how special it was to take a bite of an apple while it was still on the tree. When I was growing up, we went to various farmers' markets every harvest season and hand-picked the best tomatoes, pumpkins, cucumbers, and other vegetables. Then he made a harvest stew called Osh, a Persian, high-antioxidant, delicious, thick soup made of greens and other harvest vegetables. He was way ahead of his years and taught me that the order in which we ate food as well as the timing was as important as the food itself. We always practiced time-restricted feeding (sometimes called intermittent fasting) for a minimum of 13 hours a day. We rarely had desserts and always ate dinner as a family, making mealtime as special as the food we ate.

My mom was a great cook, and I learned that Persian meals were often packed with antioxidants such as turmeric and saffron. Then I started to study the foods of different cultures and the power of spices. My dad's best advice for a daily diet was to eat 24 almonds (about 1 ounce), 6 walnuts (high in the best fatty acids but also high in calories, so don't eat too many), at least half an avocado, no more than half a banana (high in sugar), and something green at every meal. His top recommendations were broccoli, spinach, asparagus, and fenugreek, which is very popular in Persian cooking and has many health benefits. I still follow his advice most of the time, and my skin is the better for it.

Biomes at Bedtime

Sleep is the time when all our body systems can slow down and recharge. When it comes to the skin and the skin microbiome, sleep typically happens when we are less exposed to environmental stressors such as UV radiation (unless we fall asleep at the beach, which is not advised). Sleep, or rather the lack of it, can affect the skin biome. Sleep patterns can cause the body environment to cycle throughout the 24-hour day, which in turn creates differences in the environment we provide in each of our biomes. Our circadian rhythms cause fluctuations in things such as hormones, body temperature, and blood pressure. These daily changes in our bodies are reflected in the substances our bodies produce on the skin such as the oils our skin produces, which in turn changes the overall cycles that our microbiomes follow when they reproduce or secrete certain substances. The balance of our biomes is thus achieved in coordination with our circadian rhythms. When our sleep patterns are thrown off, so is the cycle of our circadian rhythms that in turn can cause overgrowth or undergrowth of certain microbes in the biome. That can lead to undesirable changes in the skin, depending on how much dysbiosis occurs.[16]

Research suggests that dysregulation of sleep patterns can lead to increases in the creation of free radical stress in tissues. And as we have seen, there is a direct correlation with free radical stress on skin damage, including aging and cancers. When scientists have studied the effects of sleep on the skin, they have found that good sleepers tend to have less skin aging, better skin barrier recovery, and better recovery after UV damage compared to those who don't get sufficient sleep.[17]

One study that looked at those who alter their sleep patterns based on varying work shifts (sometimes day shifts, sometimes night shifts) had higher rates of psoriasis. That makes sense because less barrier repair would allow for the ingress of opportunistic pathogens on the skin. However, dysbiosis would also have to happen in order for this to occur, leading us to imagine that such phenomena have some contributing microbiome dysbiosis that may be due to circadian dysregulation.

Overall, the research to date does seem to suggest that negative metabolic changes associated with sleep loss may, in fact, be caused in part by microbial dysbiosis, in turn caused by sleep loss—a vicious cycle that involves all parts of the biome.[18] So get your beauty sleep for your skin biomes' sake.

Embracing the Biome Reboot

Dr. Hitchcock: When I was a young scientist struggling my way through graduate school to get my doctorate, I was approached by my graduate mentor about what he felt I needed to do in order to be successful. At the time I was in the third year of my doctoral studies. Not only was I doing research full time, but I was also a teaching assistant for my mentor, the president of the university's men's choir, and acting in some regional independent films and productions in the university theater program. On top of that, I was trying my hand at learning photography by which I supplemented my meager graduate student income, and I never missed a day at the gym.

My mentor had seen me perform in some of the university's concerts and plays and grew concerned that I may not be as focused as he thought I should be in order to finish my degree and become successful in my career. He was a naturalized American who worked hard after emigrating from China to the United States to get his PhD, start a family, and begin a career as a university professor. Indeed, his work ethic was impressive. Whenever I was in the lab, he was inevitably in his office, toiling tirelessly to write a grant proposal or prepare lesson plans for his classes.

One particular day, he sat me down and shared he felt that in order for me to be successful, I would need to stop doing everything except my genetics research. He referred to one of my fellow graduate students in the lab who was a year behind me and seemed to always be there from 7:00 a.m. until way after dark. The insinuation was that I should be more like that student and more like my mentor. He told me of his once avid enthusiasm for playing the guitar but that when he started graduate school, he decided not to play any longer since it was a distraction from his work—his goal.

I paused to consider what he was saying. After all, he was the professor, the mentor. But when I started to think about a life of nothing but lab work without my art or hobbies and without the welcomed respite from the stresses of the day, the prospect of what he was proposing seemed very empty and sad. You see, I had been in the lab some nights with that graduate student when the professor was not there, and I observed him not working but rather using the Internet access to video call his friends and family back home in China. It wasn't that he had a better work ethic; it was that he had nothing else to do or nowhere else to be. When I mentioned that to my professor, he retorted that I was wrong and that I'd have to put in the hours in order to be successful. Then I realized that of all the graduate students and postdoctoral candidates in the lab, I was the farthest along, I was the only one who was published, and I was the only one my mentor had required to teach while the other students got to focus solely on their research.

I realized that I did love science, but I also loved music, fitness, theater, and photography. And while there are only so many hours in the day (in retrospect, I have no idea where I got all that energy), the fact was that I was doing well in my academics and research and was actually farther along than most of the doctoral students who started with me. For me, it was the balance in my life between my work and hobbies that allowed me to function at my best. Being able to vent the stresses of my studies through my extracurricular activities was not a deterrent. It was a boon.

In the end, I defended my dissertation a year early before all my peers in the program. In my dissertation, I wrote an artsy dedication to my father, which my advisor told me I would regret. It was not the best dedication ever written, but it was my way of branding my philosophy into that chapter of my life. When I reflect on all the experiences I've had, I feel it was that time that helped shape the trajectory of my life and career the most. I learned that in order to be successful and truly happy, I had to care for myself in every aspect. I could not just foster my academic curiosities; I also had to care for my personal life, my art, my music, my spirituality, and my health. In a way, that is when my Holobiont Philosophy was born.

Dr. Day: I was an English literature major and avid athlete in college. My dad instilled in me a love of travel, and the combination of studying literature and philosophy as well as seeing the world as a student on a very tight budget taught me more about the art of medicine than all the basic science courses I would take in my post-bac years before medical school. It helped me understand the human condition and what we all have in common and it gave me the best chance at being the kind of physician I strived to be throughout my career—to understood the whole person rather than only the mechanics of illness and health and to look past what was on the surface and what was in the textbooks in order to heal patients. Adding a degree in journalism from New York University added a layer of focus on the investigative side of medicine, which came in very handy when new treatments and ideas came along, even though it delayed going to medical school by an extra few years. My father was very disappointed at the delay and did his best to dissuade me, telling me "this is the biggest mistake of your life, you will never go to medical school." He wanted me to be on a straight path and focus on my chosen career without distraction or delay. I was happy to prove him wrong and so happy to have the confidence that my education gave me to question everything I knew and to look for better ways to help my patients look and feel their best. I also wanted to focus on health and well-being, learn to investigate and question information, and then provide information in an unbiased way. It helped me recognize that our approach to skincare didn't make sense and to work on finding better ingredients and methods for treating the skin to keep it healthy as we age. Working with Thomas has been a highlight and I'm very excited for the possibilities that lie ahead. My passion and focus is on healthspan and quality of life over lifespan. My father always said, "we should all die young, at a very old age." Medicine and science is life-long learning; we are constantly building on our knowledge and have to keep an open mind that what we know as true today may change tomorrow and what we thought of as right or wrong may also change. We have to remain skeptical and always question the data, but also work and do our best with what we have and what we know now.

The Holobiont Philosophy is the realization that in order to truly care for an organism, you must care for that organism's entire ecosystem. In this book, we have outlined this very salient truth, that for the health and beauty of our skin we must adopt a lifestyle that makes sure our whole selves—human and microbiomes—are placed in the very best environment possible. That means we must examine our habits, our hygiene, our diets, our lifestyle, and our knowledge. That last one is very important, for as we discussed earlier, we can only do better if we know better.

We don't want anyone who reads these last lines of the book to think that they now have the end all and be all of what it takes to achieve the Holobiont Philosophy. Our collective wisdom is based only on what we currently know. We can't see the future. But for now, we hope the philosophy of this book will guide you to seek your own biome balance. Who knows what miracles science in medicine has in store for us in years to come?

But what we do know is that no matter how clean you think you are, you have billions of bacteria on your skin. And we think that's wonderful.

NOTES

Chapter 2

[1] Kirk R. " Life in a Germ-Free World ": Isolating Life from the Laboratory Animal to the Bubble Boy. *Bull Hist Med.* 2012;(084988):237-275.

[2] Ibid

[3] Wells HG. *The War of the World.*; 1898.

[4] R.G. The War of the Worlds. Nature. 1898;57:339-340.

[5] 10th M. Thrive without Microbes: Sterilized Guinea-Pigs Grow 30 Per Cent Faster Than Others. *New York Times.* 1914:3.

[6] Finds Life without Microbes Possible. Chickens Raised amid Microbe-Proof Conditions Just as Big and Healthy as Others in Farmyard. *New York Times.* 1912:Feb 16, pg 4 column 5.

[7] Koprowski H. Future of Infectious and Malignant Diseases. In: *Man and His Future.* Wolstenhol. ; 1963:196–216 Wolstenholme, ed.

[8] Health and Disease Discussion. In: *Man and His Future,*. ; 1963:230–46.

[9] Snyder DL, Pollard M, Wostmann BS, Luckert P. Life Span, Morphology, and Pathology of Diet-Restricted Germ-Free and Conventional Lobund-Wistar Rats. *J Gerontol.* 1990;45(2):B52-B58. doi:10.1093/geronj/45.2.B52

[10] Ibid

[11] Luczynski P, Neufeld KAMV, Oriach CS, Clarke G, Dinan TG, Cryan JF. Growing up in a bubble: Using germ-free animals to assess the influence of the gut microbiota on brain and behavior. Int J Neuropsychopharmacol. 2016;19(8):1-17. doi:10.1093/ijnp/pyw020

[12] Grenham S, Clarke G, Cryan JF, Dinan TG, Makharia GK. Brain – gut – microbe communication in health and disease. 2011;2(December):1-15. doi:10.3389/fphys.2011.00094

[13] Fischer N, Mak TN, Shinohara DB, Sfanos KS, Meyer TF, Brüggemann H. Deciphering the Intracellular Fate of Propionibacterium acnes in Macrophages. Biomed Res Int. 2013;2013:1-11. doi:10.1155/2013/603046

[14] Ibid

[15] Davidsson S, Carlsson J, Greenberg L, Wijkander J, Söderquist B, Erlandsson A. Cutibacterium acnes Induces the Expression of Immunosuppressive Genes in Macrophages and is Associated with an Increase of Regulatory T-Cells in Prostate Cancer. Claesen J, ed. *Microbiol Spectr*. 2021;9(3). doi:10.1128/spectrum.01497-21

[16] Kowarsky M, Camunas-Soler J, Kertesz M, et al. Numerous uncharacterized and highly divergent microbes which colonize humans are revealed by circulating cell-free DNA. *Proc Natl Acad Sci*. 2017;114(36):9623-9628. doi:10.1073/pnas.1707009114

[17] Sampson TR, Debelius JW, Thron T, et al. Gut Microbiota Regulate Motor Deficits and Neuroinflammation in a Model of Parkinson's Disease. *Cell*. 2016;167(6):1469-1480.e12. doi:10.1016/j.cell.2016.11.018

[18] Nielsen SD, Pearson NM, Seidler K. The link between the gut microbiota and Parkinson's Disease: A systematic mechanism review with focus on α-synuclein transport. *Brain Res*. 2021;1769:147609. doi:10.1016/j.brainres.2021.147609

[19] De Pessemier B, Grine L, Debaere M, Maes A, Paetzold B, Callewaert C. Gut–Skin Axis: Current Knowledge of the Interrelationship between Microbial Dysbiosis and Skin Conditions. *Microorganisms*. 2021;9(2):353. doi:10.3390/microorganisms9020353

[20] Martinez KA, Devlin JC, Lacher CR, et al. Increased weight gain by C-section: Functional significance of the primordial microbiome. *Sci Adv*. 2017;3(10). doi:10.1126/sciadv.aao1874

[21] Princisval L, Rebelo F, Williams BL, et al. Association Between the Mode of Delivery and Infant Gut Microbiota Composition Up to 6 Months of Age: A Systematic Literature Review Considering the Role of Breastfeeding. *Nutr Rev*. 2021;80(1):113-127. doi:10.1093/nutrit/nuab008

[22] Wang M, Radlowski EC, Monaco MH, Fahey GC, Gaskins HR, Donovan SM. Mode of delivery and early nutrition modulate microbial colonization and fermentation products in neonatal piglets. *J Nutr*. 2013;143(6):795-803. doi:10.3945/jn.112.173096

[23] Cabré S, Ratsika A, Rea K, Stanton C, Cryan JF. Animal models for assessing impact of C-section delivery on biological systems. *Neurosci Biobehav Rev*. 2022;135(February). doi:10.1016/j.neubiorev.2022.104555

[24] Jiménez E, Fernández L, Marín ML, et al. Isolation of Commensal Bacteria from Umbilical Cord Blood of Healthy Neonates Born by Cesarean Section. *Curr Microbiol.* 2005;51(4):270-274. doi:10.1007/s00284-005-0020-3

[25] Mancino W, Duranti S, Mancabelli L, et al. Bifidobacterial Transfer from Mother to Child as Examined by an Animal Model. *Microorganisms.* 2019;7(9):293. doi:10.3390/microorganisms709029

[26] Ahluwalia J, Borok J, Haddock ES, Ahluwalia RS, Schwartz EW, Hosseini D, Amini S, Eichenfield LF. The microbiome in preadolescent acne: Assessment and prospective analysis of the influence of benzoyl peroxide. Pediatr Dermatol. 2019 Mar;36(2):200-206

[27] Lam M, Hu A, Fleming P, Lynde CW. The Impact of Acne Treatment on Skin Bacterial Microbiota: A Systematic Review. J Cutan Med Surg. 2022 Jan-Feb;26(1):93-97

Chapter 3

[1] Fitz-Gibbon S, Tomida S, Chiu BH, et al. Propionibacterium acnes strain populations in the human skin microbiome associated with acne. J Invest Dermatol. 2013;133(9):2152-2160. doi:10.1038/jid.2013.21

[2] Ibid

[3] Bek-Thomsen M, Lomholt HB, Kilian M. Acne Is Not Associated with Yet-Uncultured Bacteria. J Clin Microbiol. 2008;46(10):3355-3360. doi:10.1128/JCM.00799-08

[4] Contassot E, French LE. Propionibacterium acnes Strains Differentially Regulate the Fate of Th17 Responses in the Skin. J Invest Dermatol. 2018;138(2):251-253. doi:10.1016/j.jid.2017.09.041

[5] Ibid

[6] Microbiology (2005), **151**, 1369–1379

[7] Contassot E, French LE. Propionibacterium acnes Strains Differentially Regulate the Fate of Th17 Responses in the Skin. J Invest Dermatol. 2018;138(2):251-253. doi:10.1016/j.jid.2017.09.041

[8] Andersson T, Ertürk Bergdahl G, Saleh K, et al. Common skin bacteria protect their host from oxidative stress through secreted antioxidant. RoxP. Sci Rep. 2019;9(1):3596. doi:10.1038/s41598-019-40471-3

[9] Rhee MS, Alqam ML, Jones BC, Phadungpojna S, Day D, Hitchcock TM. Characterization of a live Cutibacterium acnes subspecies defendens strain XYCM42 and clinical assessment as a topical regimen for general skin health and cosmesis. J Cosmet Dermatol. 2022 Nov 14. doi: 10.1111/jocd.15510. Epub ahead of print. PMID: 36374551.

[10] Andersson T, Ertürk Bergdahl G, Saleh K, et al. Common skin bacteria protect their host from oxidative stress through secreted antioxidant. RoxP. *Sci Rep*. 2019;9(1):3596. doi:10.1038/s41598-019-40471-3

[11] Johnson T, Kang D, Barnard E, Li H. Strain-Level Differences in Porphyrin Production and Regulation in Propionibacterium acnes Elucidate Disease Associations. D'Orazio SEF, ed. *mSphere*. 2016;1(1). doi:10.1128/mSphere.00023-15

Chapter 4

[1] Lavker RM, Leyden JJ, McGinley KJ. The Relationship between Bacteria and the Abnormal Follicular Keratinization in Acne Vulgaris. Journal of Investigative Dermatology. 1981;77(3):325-330. doi:10.1111/1523-1747.ep12482524

[2] Ibid.

[3] Luque-Ramírez M, Ortiz-Flores AE, Martínez-García MÁ, et al. Effect of Iron Depletion by Bloodletting vs. Observation on Oxidative Stress Biomarkers of Women with Functional Hyperandrogenism Taking a Combined Oral Contraceptive: A Randomized Clinical Trial. J Clin Med. 2022;11(13):3864. doi:10.3390/jcm11133864

[4] Isard O, Knol AC, Ariès MF, et al. Propionibacterium acnes Activates the IGF-1/IGF-1R System in the Epidermis and Induces Keratinocyte Proliferation. Journal of Investigative Dermatology. 2011;131(1):59-66. doi:10.1038/jid.2010.281

[5] Fitz-Gibbon S, Tomida S, Chiu BH, et al. Propionibacterium acnes Strain Populations in the Human Skin Microbiome Associated with Acne. Journal of Investigative Dermatology. 2013;133(9):2152-2160. doi:10.1038/jid.2013.21

[6] Ibid.

[7] Bowe W, Patel NB, Logan AC. Acne vulgaris, probiotics and the gut-brain-skin axis: from anecdote to translational medicine. Beneficial Microbes. 2014;5(2):185-199. doi:10.3920/BM2012.0060

[8] Okamoto K, Kanayama S, Ikeda F, Fujikawa K, Fujiwara S, Nozawa N, Mori S, Matsumoto T, Hayashi N, Oda M. Broad spectrum in vitro microbicidal activity of

benzoyl peroxide against microorganisms related to cutaneous diseases. J Dermatol. 2021 Apr;48(4):551-555. doi: 10.1111/1346-8138.15739

[9] Xu X, Ran X, Tang J, Pradhan S, Dai Y, Zhuang K, Ran Y. Skin Microbiota in Non-inflammatory and Inflammatory Lesions of Acne Vulgaris: The Underlying Changes within the Pilosebaceous Unit. Mycopathologia. 2021 Dec;186(6):863-869. doi: 10.1007/s11046-021-00586-6.) (CITE Akaza N, Takasaki K, Nishiyama E, Usui A, Miura S, Yokoi A, Futamura K, Suzuki K, Yashiro Y, Yagami A. The Microbiome in Comedonal Contents of Inflammatory Acne Vulgaris is Composed of an Overgrowth of Cutibacterium Spp. and Other Cutaneous Microorganisms. Clin Cosmet Investig Dermatol. 2022 Sep 21;15:2003-2012. doi: 10.2147/CCID.S379609. PMID: 36172249; PMCID: PMC9510696

[10] Lavker RM, Leyden JJ, McGinley KJ. The Relationship between Bacteria and the Abnormal Follicular Keratinization in Acne Vulgaris. Journal of Investigative Dermatology. 1981;77(3):325-330. doi:10.1111/1523-1747.ep12482524

[11] Boguniewicz M, Leung DYM. Atopic dermatitis: a disease of altered skin barrier and immune dysregulation. Immunological Reviews. 2011;242(1):233-246. doi:10.1111/j.1600-065X.2011.01027.x

[12] Garmhausen D, Hagemann T, Bieber T, et al. Characterization of different courses of atopic dermatitis in adolescent and adult patients. Allergy. 2013;68(4):498-506. doi:10.1111/all.12112

[13] Shaw TE, Currie GP, Koudelka CW, Simpson EL. Eczema Prevalence in the United States: Data from the 2003 National Survey of Children's Health. Journal of Investigative Dermatology. 2011;131(1):67-73. doi:10.1038/jid.2010.251

[14] Silverberg JI, Garg NK, Paller AS, Fishbein AB, Zee PC. Sleep Disturbances in Adults with Eczema Are Associated with Impaired Overall Health: A US Population-Based Study. Journal of Investigative Dermatology. 2015;135(1):56-66. doi:10.1038/jid.2014.325

[15] McLean WHI, Palmer CNA, Henderson J, Kabesch M, Weidinger S, Irvine AD. Filaggrin variants confer susceptibility to asthma. Journal of Allergy and Clinical Immunology. 2008;121(5):1294-1295. doi:10.1016/j.jaci.2008.02.039

[16] Boguniewicz M, Leung DYM. Atopic dermatitis: a disease of altered skin barrier and immune dysregulation. Immunological Reviews. 2011;242(1):233-246. doi:10.1111/j.1600-065X.2011.01027.x

[17] Ibid.

[18] Garmhausen D, Hagemann T, Bieber T, et al. Characterization of different courses of atopic dermatitis in adolescent and adult patients. Allergy. 2013;68(4):498-506. doi:10.1111/all.12112

[19] Bieber T. Interleukin-13: Targeting an underestimated cytokine in atopic dermatitis. Allergy. 2020;75(1):54-62. doi:10.1111/all.13954

[20] Zhang E, Tanaka T, Tajima M, Tsuboi R, Nishikawa A, Sugita T. Characterization of the skin fungal microbiota in patients with atopic dermatitis and in healthy subjects. Microbiology and Immunology. 2011;55(9):625-632. doi:10.1111/j.1348-0421.2011.00364.x

[21] Gonzalez ME, Schaffer J v., Orlow SJ, et al. Cutaneous microbiome effects of fluticasone propionate cream and adjunctive bleach baths in childhood atopic dermatitis. Journal of the American Academy of Dermatology. 2016;75(3):481-493.e8. doi:10.1016/j.jaad.2016.04.066

[22] Ibid.

[23] Iwamoto K, Moriwaki M, Miyake R, Hide M. Staphylococcus aureus in atopic dermatitis: Strain-specific cell wall proteins and skin immunity. Allergology International. 2019;68(3):309-315. doi:10.1016/j.alit.2019.02.006

[24] Byrd AL, Deming C, Cassidy SKB, et al. Staphylococcus aureus and Staphylococcus epidermidis strain diversity underlying pediatric atopic dermatitis. Science Translational Medicine. 2017;9(397). doi:10.1126/scitranslmed.aal4651

[25] Clausen ML, Agner T, Lilje B, Edslev SM, Johannesen TB, Andersen PS. Association of Disease Severity With Skin Microbiome and Filaggrin Gene Mutations in Adult Atopic Dermatitis. JAMA Dermatology. 2018;154(3):293. doi:10.1001/jamadermatol.2017.5440

[26] Nakatsuji T, Chen TH, Narala S, et al. Antimicrobials from human skin commensal bacteria protect against Staphylococcus aureus and are deficient in atopic dermatitis. Science Translational Medicine. 2017;9(378). doi:10.1126/scitranslmed.aah4680

[27] Wood DLA, Lachner N, Tan JM, et al. A Natural History of Actinic Keratosis and Cutaneous Squamous Cell Carcinoma Microbiomes. mBio. 2018;9(5). doi:10.1128/mBio.01432-18

[28] Chen YE, Tsao H. The skin microbiome: Current perspectives and future challenges. Journal of the American Academy of Dermatology. 2013;69(1):143-155.e3. doi:10.1016/j.jaad.2013.01.016

[29] Beachy PA, Karhadkar SS, Berman DM. Tissue repair and stem cell renewal in carcinogenesis. Nature. 2004;432(7015):324-331. doi:10.1038/nature03100

[30] Ibid.

[31] Zhang M, Qureshi AA, Fortner RT, et al. Teenage acne and cancer risk in US women: A prospective cohort study. Cancer. 2015;121(10):1681-1687. doi:10.1002/cncr.29216

[32] Ibid.

[33] Sherwani MA, Tufail S, Muzaffar AF, Yusuf N. The skin microbiome and immune system: Potential target for chemoprevention? Photodermatology, Photoimmunology & Photomedicine. 2018;34(1):25-34. doi:10.1111/phpp.12334

[34] Burns EM, Yusuf N. Toll-Like Receptors and Skin Cancer. Frontiers in Immunology. 2014;5. doi:10.3389/fimmu.2014.00135

[35] Ibid.

Chapter 7

[1] Capone K, Kirchner F, Klein SL, Tierney NK. Effects of Colloidal Oatmeal Topical Atopic Dermatitis Cream on Skin Microbiome and Skin Barrier Properties. J Drugs Dermatol. 2020 May 1;19(5):524-531. PMID: 32484623.

Chapter 8

[1] Bertone MA, Leong M, Bayless KM, Malow TLF, Dunn RR, Trautwein MD. Arthropods of the great indoors: characterizing diversity inside urban and suburban homes. *PeerJ*. 2016;4:e1582. doi:10.7717/peerj.1582

[2] Proksch E, Brandner JM, Jensen J-M. The skin: an indispensable barrier. Exp Dermatol. 2008;17(12):1063-1072. doi:10.1111/j.1600-0625.2008.00786.x

[3] Biniek K, Levi K, Dauskardt RH. Solar UV radiation reduces the barrier function of human skin. *Proc Natl Acad Sci*. 2012;109(42):17111-17116. doi:10.1073/pnas.1206851109

[4] Widhiati S, Purnomosari D, Wibawa T, Soebono H. The role of gut microbiome in inflammatory skin disorders: a systematic review. *Dermatology Reports*. Published online December 28, 2021. doi:10.4081/dr.2022.9188

[5] De Pessemier B, Grine L, Debaere M, Maes A, Paetzold B, Callewaert C. Gut–Skin Axis: Current Knowledge of the Interrelationship between Microbial Dysbiosis and

Skin Conditions. *Microorganisms*. 2021;9(2):353. doi:10.3390/microorganisms9020353

⁶ Mahmud MR, Akter S, Tamanna SK, et al. Impact of gut microbiome on skin health: gut-skin axis observed through the lenses of therapeutics and skin diseases. *Gut Microbes*. 2022;14(1). doi:10.1080/19490976.2022.2096995

⁷ Szlachcic A. The link between Helicobacter pylori infection and rosacea. *J Eur Acad Dermatology Venereol*. 2002;16(4):328-333. doi:10.1046/j.1468-3083.2002.00497.x

⁸ Holscher HD. Dietary fiber and prebiotics and the gastrointestinal microbiota. *Gut Microbes*. 2017;8(2):172-184. doi:10.1080/19490976.2017.1290756

⁹ Deehan EC, Walter J. The Fiber Gap and the Disappearing Gut Microbiome: Implications for Human Nutrition. *Trends Endocrinol Metab*. 2016;27(5):239-242. doi:10.1016/j.tem.2016.03.001

¹⁰ Baldwin H, Tan J. Effects of Diet on Acne and Its Response to Treatment. *Am J Clin Dermatol*. 2021;22(1):55-65. doi:10.1007/s40257-020-00542-y

Chapter 9

¹ Iheozor-Ejiofor Z, Worthington H V, Walsh T, et al. Water fluoridation for the prevention of dental caries. Cochrane Database Syst Rev. Published online June 18, 2015. doi:10.1002/14651858.CD010856.pub2

² Choi AL, Sun G, Zhang Y, Grandjean P. Developmental Fluoride Neurotoxicity: A Systematic Review and Meta-Analysis. Environ Health Perspect. 2012;120(10):1362-1368. doi:10.1289/ehp.1104912

³ Chassaing B, Koren O, Goodrich JK, et al. Dietary emulsifiers impact the mouse gut microbiota promoting colitis and metabolic syndrome. *Nature*. 2015;519(7541):92-96. doi:10.1038/nature14232

⁴ Suez J, Korem T, Zeevi D, et al. Artificial sweeteners induce glucose intolerance by altering the gut microbiota. *Nature*. 2014;514(7521):181-186. doi:10.1038/nature13793

⁵ Li P, Li M, Wu T, et al. Systematic evaluation of antimicrobial food preservatives on glucose metabolism and gut microbiota in healthy mice. *npj Sci Food*. 2022;6(1):42. doi:10.1038/s41538-022-00158-y

⁶ Biniek K, Levi K, Dauskardt RH. Solar UV radiation reduces the barrier function of human skin. Proc Natl Acad Sci. 2012;109(42):17111-17116. doi:10.1073/pnas.1206851109

[7] Kollias N. The Absorption Properties of "Physical" Sunscreens. Arch Dermatol. 1999;135(2):209-a-210. doi:10.1001/archderm.135.2.209-a

[8] Cole C, Shyr T, Ou-Yang H. Metal oxide sunscreens protect skin by absorption, not by reflection or scattering. Photodermatol Photoimmunol Photomed. 2016;32(1):5-10. doi:10.1111/phpp.12214

[9] Neale RE, Khan SR, Lucas RM, Waterhouse M, Whiteman DC, Olsen CM. The effect of sunscreen on vitamin D: a review. Br J Dermatol. 2019;181(5):907-915. doi:10.1111/bjd.17980

[10] Ibid.

[11] Lipner SR. Reply to: "Response to 'Rethinking biotin therapy for hair, nail, and skin disorders.'" J Am Acad Dermatol. 2018;79(6):e125. doi:10.1016/j.jaad.2018.08.002

[12] Ibid.

[13] Holscher HD. Dietary fiber and prebiotics and the gastrointestinal microbiota. Gut Microbes. 2017;8(2):172-184. doi:10.1080/19490976.2017.1290756

[14] Deehan EC, Walter J. The Fiber Gap and the Disappearing Gut Microbiome: Implications for Human Nutrition. Trends Endocrinol Metab. 2016;27(5):239-242. doi:10.1016/j.tem.2016.03.001

[15] Baldwin H, Tan J. Effects of Diet on Acne and Its Response to Treatment. Am J Clin Dermatol. 2021;22(1):55-65. doi:10.1007/s40257-020-00542-y

[16] Matsui M, Pelle E, Dong K, Pernodet N. Biological Rhythms in the Skin. Int J Mol Sci. 2016;17(6):801. doi:10.3390/ijms17060801

[17] Oyetakin-White P, Suggs A, Koo B, et al. Does poor sleep quality affect skin ageing? *Clin Exp Dermatol.* 2015;40(1):17-22. doi:10.1111/ced.12455

[18] Matenchuk BA, Mandhane PJ, Kozyrskyj AL. Sleep, circadian rhythm, and gut microbiota. *Sleep Med Rev.* 2020;53:101340. doi:10.1016/j.smrv.2020.101340

Printed in Poland
by Amazon Fulfillment
Poland Sp. z o.o., Wrocław
03 November 2023